THE
LATINA
ANTI-DIET

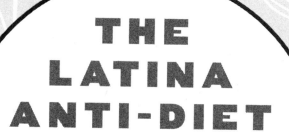

THE LATINA ANTI-DIET

A DIETITIAN'S GUIDE TO AUTHENTIC HEALTH THAT CELEBRATES CULTURE AND FULL-FLAVOR LIVING

DALINA SOTO,
MA, RD, LDN

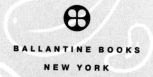

BALLANTINE BOOKS

NEW YORK

Published in the United States by Ballantine Books, an imprint of Random House, a division of Penguin Random House LLC, 1745 Broadway, New York, NY 10019.

BALLANTINE BOOKS & colophon are registered trademarks of Penguin Random House LLC.

Hardcover ISBN 978-0-593-72622-8
Ebook ISBN 978-0-593-72623-5

Printed in the United States of America on acid-free paper

randomhousebooks.com
penguinrandomhouse.com

1st Printing

First Edition

Book design by Jo Anne Metsch

The authorized representative in the EU for product safety and compliance is Penguin Random House Ireland, Morrison Chambers, 32 Nassau Street, Dublin D02 YH68, Ireland. https://eu-contact.penguin.ie

To ALL of us who have been told by society we aren't enough and that we need to change who we are to fit a mold that was never created for us. We are enough y punto.

CONTENTS

INTRODUCTION

I F you step through the heavy front door of an old building in the Bronx, you'll immediately be greeted by small, checkered white-and-black tiles and brown walls. The halls smell musty, and nostalgia for the 1980s and '90s seeps through the walls. Mi abuela lived on the second floor of one of these buildings on Union Avenue, while my parents and I lived on the first floor of that same building, right underneath her. My mom says I knew the sound of mi abuela's footsteps, and that she could not step one foot downstairs without me screaming for her to pick me up, play with me, give me attention. Mi abuela was brilliant; I am here today because of her.

Many say I get my stubbornness from her, which I consider a great compliment. She took *zero* shit, and she came to the United States to provide a better life for her kids. My mom is the youngest of eight. She was the first to land in Nueva York, and soon after, I arrived as the first American-born grandchild.

Sometimes, I can still smell mi abuela. I remember her always cooking and singing in her kitchen, full of joy for what she had provided for her family, a new beginning. When she left the Dominican Republic, things were not good. Rafael Trujillo, a horrible dictator, had been assassinated literally the day after my dad was born in 1961. The country was still in a shambles almost a decade later when mi abuela decided to come to the United States to build a better life for her eight children, who stayed behind in the Dominican Republic while she pursued the American Dream for their futures.

I didn't live in the Bronx for long. My parents moved around before landing in Philadelphia when I was three, but being only an hour and a half away meant we spent a lot of time in the Bronx with mi abuela. She had a small two-bedroom apartment that my cousins, siblings, family friends, and I all crammed into during the summers. I grew up playing on the fire escapes and getting wet in the torrents of water from open fire hydrants. We spent carefree years playing and running through those halls, never having to use the elevator, which barely worked anyway. At one point my tía lived in the apartment next to my abuela, and I remember all of us kids laughing, running back and forth between the two apartments for parties and food. My primos introduced me to Biggie's music on the steps of that Bronx building, and I vividly remember being in a taxi driving back from shopping on la tercera, Third Avenue, when we found out Aaliyah had passed away. Fun fact: I also discovered my love for Aventura because Romeo Santos went to South Bronx High School with my primos and they gifted me the Aventura CD he used to pass around at school. Damn, I wish I still had that.

If you grew up in New York City, you know bodegas were on every corner, sometimes at both ends of the block, each selling the same thing, but you always had a favorite anyway. My primos, brothers, and I grew up so carefree. We would eat freely from the bodegas (they kept running tabs for our parents), and sugar and "junk food" were not things we thought about. We spent hours running up and down the block, hanging from the fire escapes, and watching adults dancing to bachata and merengue while we ran in and out of the fire hydrants' spray. How I wish my kids could experience this pure joy, with no tablets, no phones, no social media.

Growing up, food was everything. I grew up eating *all* the Dominican foods because I am Dominican, first generation and proud. For my family, Dominican food was *the* food, and there was always comida en casa—I mean *always*.

I have so many memories of mi abuela's food, of her cooking locrio, moro, sancocho, and arroz con leche, of us taking turns on the kitchen stool to taste the food or help her cook. Mi abuela loved to cook, and she was amazing at it. She always fed us and we all ate the same exact things. There was rarely any talk about bodies—we were all equal in her eyes. And to be honest, looking back, I think this is why I questioned if diet culture was a real thing when I was just starting in my dietetics journey. We ate the same, ran the same, drank all the sodas and frambuesa Country Clubs (IYKYK), and yet we were different. We all ate arroz con habichuelas daily, we all drank jugos, we all just *ate*.

I was thin, or "normal" as many adults would say now, and I was never forced to clean my plate. I mean, did I hear "There are hungry children in Santo Domingo wishing they had a warm plate of food"? Yes, often, as we all did. But I was never forced to finish every single thing on my plate just for the heck of it. In the eyes of my family, I didn't need to be controlled around food, and neither did any of my primas. Maybe we were just ahead of our time as a family, but I know that's not the case for many, especially in the Latine community, where many grow up hearing that they have to eat more while being expected to not get bigger. It was and still is such a mindfuck, this idea that you must eat all the food on your plate and bypass your fullness cues but never, ever, *ever* gain weight.

Health wasn't something that was emphasized in my family because we knew what we were eating was healthy. Besides the snack tab at the bodega, we rarely ate out, not because it was considered "bad" but because someone was always cooking and feeding everyone on the block. To this day, I still believe that our cultural foods are the best. Rice, beans, meat, and cabbage salad were the staples of my existence then, and still are now. That complete meal nourished me daily, and now it nourishes my kids (except for the cabbage, which my kids are currently boycotting). And if you have a Latina mom, I know you get that daily phone call to see what you fed your kids—and that you get an earful if it wasn't something up to her standards.

Growing up, I always felt I was allowed to just *be*. While comments were never explicitly made about my body, body image was something I struggled with in a different way, not because of my family (which I know is the case for many Latino families), but because of TV. If you grew up watching telenovelas, you know the gold standard was very European looks. The leading ladies never looked a thing like me, and let's be honest, we *all* wanted the flat belly, small waist, and long-ass hair. Some of y'all might have had that, but I didn't. My hair was wildly curly, so I straightened it weekly to fit in. My nickname for years was panza de maco, which translated from Dominican means "belly like a frog." This nickname went away once my teenage years came along and my potbelly disappeared, but it wasn't until I was an adult that I realized how much it had affected me.

However, unlike many others growing up in a Latine family, this nickname never changed the way I ate or acted. As with many nicknames, you don't get to choose them, they are usually very inappropriate, and they never go away. Luckily for me my nickname did disappear eventually; the fact that I wanted a flatter belly never did. I am not sure if it's because of my lack of giving a shit about things like that or that I had thin privilege (even though I didn't have the words for it yet), but I truly never tried to alter my eating habits to change my belly. It went away on its own, but I recognize that's not the case for everyone.

I never reached the point where I wanted to change my body by doing anything extreme. When I started my university studies, I was confronted by the reality that people around me did. This was the first time I was around more thin and white people than I had ever been around in my life, and I saw people restrict their food choices and talk about their bodies in a way I had never experienced.

Like many first-gen Americans, I went to college with the hope of making my parents proud as the first one in my family to graduate from a university. I started my journey at Pennsylvania State University in 2006 as a pre-med major, and ya girl wanted to be a pediatrician. In my freshman year, my adviser told me I needed to add one more credit in phys ed to my fall semester as part of the scholarship I'd gotten to go to Penn State. But, in typical Dalina fashion, as someone who hated sports and physical activity, I dragged my feet signing up for a phys ed credit in time. Because I waited so long, I ended up in Nutrition 101 to satisfy the requirements of my scholarship.

This is where my love of nutrition started. I had always loved food, but I'd never realized it has such an important role in health. I never truly saw food as "medicine." Food was just food, but when I took this class, my perspective changed. Immediately, I decided that I wanted to become a registered dietitian. That semester taught me that I did not want to wait until people were sick to help them, I wanted to help them beforehand. I knew I wanted to use my passion for science to make a difference in my community.

And that's what I set out to do. Little did I know that the lack of diversity in the field, the misconceptions about Latine foods, and social determinants were the real factors responsible for keeping my Latino communities sick. I was taught a very whitewashed nutrition that led to a lot of dissonance between knowing who I wanted to serve but not knowing what kind of dietitian I wanted to be.

I created my social media account in 2018 and called it Nutritiously Yours, the name of my private practice in Philadelphia. I did not consistently post content, and I was not clear yet on my content niche. But in 2019, I was trying to expand my practice and so freaking frustrated by the misinformation about nutrition out in the world, and specifically in the Latine community, and I was ready to take things seriously. I was already seeing patients with insurance in person, but I wanted to expand into online counseling, so I worked with a business coach to set up that part of my practice. She urged me to change my Instagram handle to something people could connect with, and I knew exactly what it needed to be. Your.Latina.Nutritionist was born.

People who started following me were ready to hear a different perspective on nutrition, and they stuck around for the sass, real-life viewpoints, and cursing. You may be wondering why I chose Your.Latina.Nutritionist and not Your.Latina.Dietitian since I am a registered dietitian. One reason is that most people have no clue what a dietitian is, while a nutritionist is a bit more commonly known.

Secondly, it's important to point out that while all dietitians are nutritionists, not all nutritionists are dietitians, because nutritionist is not a licensed term. Dietitians have at minimum a bachelor's degree in nutritional sciences. I went to Penn State (*WE ARE*), where I completed 1,200 hours of supervised practice (aka an unpaid internship or "residency") and then sat for my registration exam to become a registered dietitian. We learned how to tube-feed people, treat disease with nutrition, and counsel patients (although we can always get more training in this, in my opinion). I wanted to become a better counselor, so I got my master's degree in nutrition education. A new requirement of the Academy of Nutrition and Dietetics is that by 2025, all new registered dietitians will need a master's degree. But anyone can call themselves a nutritionist because it's not a monitored term. So before working with someone, please check their credentials to make sure they're registered with the Commission on Dietetic Registration, the credentialing arm of the Academy of Nutrition and Dietetics. There are a lot of people who only take a three-hour course and call themselves professionals.

I decided to write this book because I recognized that many of the people I work with and speak to daily have no idea how healthy our cultural foods can be. I want to challenge these narratives, and I want to uplift notions that you can pursue nutrition with a positive lens.

While I firmly believe that anyone reading this will be able to take away valuable information for their journey to food freedom, I want to emphasize that this book will focus on Latine food and culture. Throughout the book, I will be using the word "Latine" to describe cultural foods. Latine is the gender-neutral term that is more easily pronounced than Latinx in the native Spanish tongue. I might use Latinx here and there depending on how my fingers type, but they both mean the same. As for me, I describe myself as a Latina, and I lovingly call my followers chulas. "Chula" is a term of endearment, and I kind of just started using it in posts on IG and people loved it, and boom, it stuck. As we dive into this book together, you'll have the opportunity to see yourself in other chulas' stories. I believe all people deserve to be treated with dignity and respect regardless of their gender identity, sex, or race.

And although this book is meant to teach all, I will be speaking from my Latina experience, which might not fit your particular experience as someone who is Latine, Latina, Latinx, BIPOC, or white, and that is okay.

I AM GOING to be hella honest and vulnerable with you all: Writing a damn book is hard. I want to get it right, I want my community to feel seen and heard. I don't want more stereotypes about us. I want us to be celebrated, which means I need to write a book that we deserve. That puts a lot of pressure on me because imposter syndrome sneaks in and tells me that I am not good enough and that I am going to fuck up. I recognize that my message won't resonate with everyone, but my hope is that there is something here that you can take away to improve your own relationship with food.

The truth is, I live in a thin body, and I benefit from thin privilege. It's important to acknowledge that talking about diet culture and weight while I do not deal with the day-to-day violence against fat bodies often feels wrong to me. I know that even though my body mass index (BMI) classifies me as "overweight," I can walk into a doctor's office and not a single word will be said about my weight. I know that I have the privilege of being seen by the medical world as healthy because I present as thin, and that not many people will question me about my weight (well, some trolls call me names). And I know how hard it is to experience the opposite, so I am not here to tell you how to feel, because that's just fucking wrong.

If we truly want to dismantle diet culture, which is the same as the patriarchy, which is the same as white supremacy, we have a lot of work to do. I do not have all the lived experiences, but as a registered dietitian, I will use my privileges to spread this information and help in the ways I can to educate others about food and health. I will speak about these issues and elevate those voices that I can and be honest with you all. I was once told by a nurse practitioner, "I am not an addict; I do not have that lived experience. Yet I listen to my patients, hold space for them, and do what I can to help them. I do not need to be an addict to be their nurse. You don't need to be fat or have that lived experience to help people feel seen and to do this work."

This book is for people in bigger bodies so they feel seen and heard, *not judged or shamed*. As a dietitian, my job is to help people become healthier—whatever that means for them.

This is not a weight-loss book. This book is about nutrition and healing our relationship with food. That said, I do not shame people for wanting to lose weight—who the fuck doesn't? Society has told us we need to be thin to be pretty, thin to be accepted, thin to just be treated with dignity and respect. And that fucking sucks. All we can do is try to find peace and stability with our weight.

This book creates a place where you, your comida, and your cultura are seen. It might not hit every single point beneath the health and nutrition umbrella, and that is okay. It should not be taken as gospel, because that's how shit goes sideways (I see you, Intuitive Eating movement). So, as you are reading, know that I am trying my best with the knowledge I have right now, and that the more I learn, the more I undo the problematic ideals I have been taught. I urge you to continue learning from fat liberationists. I do not have the lived experience of someone in a larger body, so I implore you to seek out the amazing fat liberationists who are sharing their work and stories and learn from them. Listen to them. They are putting in the work and should be recognized.

I hope to elevate my community, and for the most part, I will be using stories of women, my chulas, who have worked with me.

I will call out racism, white supremacy, fatphobia, homophobia, transphobia, and all other issues that can affect someone's access to food and health. If these issues make you uncomfortable, maybe this isn't the book for you. And that is quite all right. I know I am not everyone's cup of cafecito.

Although I am a registered dietitian, I want to note that I am not *your* dietitian. What you'll read in this book are very generalized guidelines, and you should always consult with your medical professionals for individualized care.

Throughout this book, I'm going to show you how diet culture has become so ingrained in our society. Even though the word "diet" has taken on a more negative connotation in recent years, it still manages to infiltrate every aspect of our culture. I'll teach you about the good things the Intuitive Eating movement has done to challenge diet culture, as well as where it fails to cater to our culture and why it's important to center our cultural foods. I'll share my guide to achieving authentic health through my CHULA Method. One size can never fit all when it comes to health, but my hope is to give you the tools you need to make decisions that work for *you*.

I am writing this book for those who, like me, grew up listening to 2000s old-school reggaeton, who spent many nights perreando to Don Omar and Wisin y Yandel. Who blasted Daddy Yankee's "Gasolina." Who would do absolutely anything to meet Romeo Santos (ROMEO, I LOVE YOU!!). And for any Latina who has been personally victimized by the words "Mija, estas gorda."

This book is for those who are tired of being told that our Latine foods are bad, that we should stop eating tortillas, and that brown rice is better than white rice. (Spoiler alert: It's *not*.)

This book is so you can feel seen and heard. As a Latina, I know the culture, I know the traditions, I eat the foods. I know the science too, and I want to bring it to you in a way that will help you heal not only *your* relationship with food, but also your mami's, your prima's, your tía's. I hope that together we can break free of generational traumas and learn to truly embrace our full selves.

My biggest fear is that diet culture will steal our traditions and we will no longer have them to pass down to our kids. I want my kids to grow up eating the foods my mami taught me to make, and I hope they will teach their kids, because food is so much more than just calories. Food is love. Food is tradition.

My hope is that after you read this book, you'll just eat: Eat with joy, eat for health, eat without fear.

TLDR: My name is Dalina. I am a first-gen Dominicana and I have two amazing kiddos. I love nutrition. I know and have the science to back up the fact that our cultural foods are amazing. No, we don't need to change them! And everyone, and I mean *everyone*, deserves to be treated with dignity and respect. I am going to teach you to heal your relationship with food in this book. Let's do this shit, chula!

PART ONE

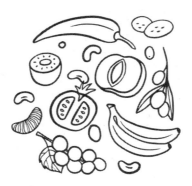

1

LAS DIETAS AND YOU

Chula Story: Vanessa

VANESSA is a twenty-seven-year-old living in L.A., where she works as a schoolteacher. She found me on Instagram and began working with me a year after her doctor told her that she was "obese" and needed to lose weight. No matter how good the results that came back from her lab work, they always pushed her to lose weight, saying that if she didn't change her ways, she would most certainly become diabetic because of her BMI. Her doctor told her that the Mexican food she was eating was "bad" and that because she was eating rice and tortillas, she had a 50 percent chance of becoming diabetic.

In a panic, Vanessa did what anyone would do: She started a diet. She first began dieting when she was fifteen, in preparation for her quinceañera, and her participation in diets continued into her adulthood. This is a story that many of you know: starting a diet for a specific reason, only to have to repeat the cycle again later on.

And in this case, Vanessa was asked by her doctor to diet again. She cut out all Mexican foods, began counting calories, and soon became obsessed. She could not stop thinking about food and calories and "earning" what she ate. As many people do when they go on rigorous diets, she lost weight, but her friends started noticing how preoccupied she was and became worried. Her hair was thinning, her nails were brittle, and she barely ate and spent all her time at the gym.

To many this seems "healthy"—she was constantly being told how amazing she looked and how much willpower she had. The constant reassurance kept her wanting to keep going. A year later, she went back to the doctor and was told that everything she had done was not enough because her BMI was still not normal. Throughout this chapter, we will follow Vanessa's story to discuss how diet culture was created and how weight stigma within the medical system can cause more harm than good.

DISMANTLING DIET CULTURE

Before we can discuss the steps we can take on our journey to achieve food freedom, we first need to look at what has negatively impacted our relationship with food in the first place. And the primary suspect is diet culture.

Diet culture is a societal belief system that values and promotes the idea that intentional weight loss, thinness, and restrictive eating is the only way to achieve health and well-being. This belief system has been heavily perpetuated by Western media and capitalism, as I will show throughout this chapter. When I search "healthy eating" in my Instagram search bar at the time of this writing, I am inundated with images and videos that primarily emphasize weight loss, low calorie swaps, meals for staying full while cutting calories, and body composition.

This system of beliefs makes us feel inferior, like we need to change and that everything about our cultures, our looks, and our bodies is wrong. It instills fear that if we are not thin, we are not healthy. If we are not restricting, we are not healthy, and if we are not eating like a white woman, you guessed it, we are not healthy.

It's pretty clear that our society is obsessed with thinness, and this obsession stems from more than one place, including beliefs in the medical community and the media's perpetuation of beauty standards. In associating thinness with goodness and social acceptance, society pressures all of us to feel like we need to be thin to be considered worthy. And as you'll see, that's a slippery slope that many of us can fall down.

BMI IS BULLSHIT!

I am sure Vanessa's story resonated with many of you, and I am sure many of you have been personally victimized by BMI. BMI is an acronym for "body mass index." The formula used to calculate BMI is the medical system's favorite little equation to supposedly figure out health. But as many before me have pointed out, it isn't an accurate measure of health, and it was never intended to be. I personally define it as an equation that uses our height and weight to determine if we are worthy of being treated with dignity and respect by the medical system. The truth is that many of us have probably been told we are in a higher-than-normal BMI category, and that's made us feel like utter shit. Let's break down the history and the ridiculousness behind this little equation.

The basis for BMI was created in the 1830s by Adolphe Quetelet, a Belgian mathematician, statistician, and sociologist. He was on a mission to define the "normal" man representing the population and "ideal" beauty. The formula uses your weight in kilograms divided by your height in meters squared. Quetelet himself did not think it should be used for individuals, but rather for populations—after all, he was a statistician.[1] Quetelet cofounded the school of positivist criminology, a doctrine that laid the groundwork for eugenics, which was an ideology that had begun popping up in the late nineteenth century. Eugenics is the "science" of improving human genetics through various interventions (does this sound eerily similar to the wellness world of today?). For example, Italian criminologist and doctor Cesare Lombroso theorized that a person with "marks of degeneration" was more likely to commit crimes. In other words, an individual's appearance, such as the shape of their cheeks or the size of their ears, was used to gauge their dangerousness. While Lombroso's theory of atavism is largely rejected, I find it important to share that different researchers in this time period, from the mid-1800s to the early 1900s, emphasized physical characteristics to a point of dehumanizing them.[2] Basically, white men used BMI to identify what bodies were (and still are) considered ideal and beautiful while pathologizing and trying to erase undesirable characteristics and disabilities to better the white race.

Many will argue that BMI itself was not created to be racist. But the thing is, BMI was conceptualized during a time when prevailing attitudes labeled people of color—specifically Black people—as "savages" and white individuals as the "ideal" of beauty. At the time, people who looked like the global majority weren't technically viewed as people, so saying BMI wasn't explicitly created to be racist erases the fact that Black people were dehumanized based on their appearance. And this remains true today.

BMI became a method of determining ideal health as early as 1895 with the introduction of a height-and-weight table that became a life-insurance industry standard. By the 1940s, a tool that was intended for standardization in developing life-insurance policies became a new standard on its own for identifying ideal body weights in the medical field. In the 1950s, doctors started using these charts to determine the "desirable weight" of their patients. To this day, BMI is used by both medical providers and insurance companies. While the Affordable Care Act prohibits insurance companies from using BMI as a factor to approve or deny coverage, it is not uncommon for folks in larger bodies to be delayed medical procedures until they've lost weight first.

Then Ancel Keys, an American physiologist who studied primarily diets and heart disease, decided to take a fresh look at determining what was a "healthy" weight. In 1972, he published a paper reporting on his comparisons of different anthropometric methods of measuring body fat. In this particular paper, Keys analyzed data from about 7,500 middle-aged men from the United States, Japan, Italy, Finland, and South Africa. (Note that this one study, even with a large sample size, includes young and older working men, without much diversity for race or class.)[3] After this study, more researchers started to use Keys's weight-divided-by-height-squared formula, and the term "body mass index" was coined.[4] Then, in 1985, the National Institutes of Health (NIH) began to use BMI categories in its definitions of "overweight" and "obesity." The World Health Organization (WHO) adopted BMI in the early 1990s.

The current categories are as follows:*

If your BMI is < 18.5 kg/m², it falls within the underweight range.

---

* You will notice throughout the text that I put certain terms, like "obesity," in quotation marks to acknowledge that the word can mean different things to different people. Use of these terms can be very pathologizing to those who live in larger bodies. However, they are used in the medical and scientific world, so when I am citing research or data, the words will be included, but always in quotation marks.

If your BMI is 18.5 to < 25 kg/m², it falls within the healthy weight range.

If your BMI is 25 to < 30 kg/m², it falls within the "overweight" range.

If your BMI is 30 kg/m² or higher, it falls within the "obesity" range.

Before 1998, the NIH classified a BMI of 18.5 to less than 27.8 for men and less than 27.3 for women as normal, but in that year the upper limit for that category was reduced for all people to less than 25, making nearly thirty million Americans overweight or obese overnight. That stirred up a lot of controversy. This decision was made to streamline the BMI classifications, but the change in the categorization of millions of people had a medical and social impact. The impact I'm talking about is weight stigma, which we will discuss later in this chapter.[5]

But first, let's talk about why BMI harms us more than it helps us find "health":

1. It oversimplifies health and does not measure fat versus muscle, the distribution of fat, bone density, or overall health.
2. It does not account for differences in body composition by age, sex, ethnicity, or social determinants of health, all of which can impact a person's health.
3. It reinforces weight stigma, making healthcare professionals focus too much on weight as a result of behavior and overlook other indicators of disease; they therefore neglect to have conversations that can identify the main problems or cause them to take the symptoms seriously.
4. It can lead to harmful dieting behaviors and disordered eating patterns, such as weight cycling, in the pursuit of a "healthy"

BMI. These are detrimental to your health and increase your risk for chronic conditions more than a higher BMI category ever will.

Because there are categorized healthy and unhealthy BMIs, BMI pathologizes the individual. This "diagnosis" can lead a person to begin a pursuit of health by focusing solely on weight rather than health-promoting behaviors. This puts a person at risk of developing disordered eating habits. This type of "health" is really healthism, which is a belief that every individual should be "textbook healthy" all the time, no matter what, as a moral obligation. According to this line of thinking, to not pursue health for your individual self is morally reprehensible.

As you can imagine, this is not true whatsoever. First, some people are born with genetic issues that don't allow them to be "textbook healthy," and second, even when they do everything right, some people still get sick. Healthism hurts us all. It places excessive focus on health and can lead to discrimination such as weight stigma, exclusion of those with disabilities or chronic illnesses, and pressuring people to go on unsustainable diets.

With the interplay of purity and diet cultures alongside our societal pressure to achieve the thin ideal, we can be left with complicated feelings about health. We are made to feel that we are a burden to society for occupying larger bodies and that we are lazy for living in larger bodies. Due to this, we may also find that as we pursue thinness, we experience greater privilege and treatment from others, including medical providers. When we're told "good job" or "congratulations" for losing weight without solicitation, we are reminded over and over again that it is a good thing to lose weight and thus a bad thing to gain weight. We have to remember that losing weight is not inherently a behavior or a pursuit of health, and we do not owe anyone that pursuit of health in order to achieve fair treatment. And yet healthism makes it very clear that the only way anyone is worthy is if they are healthy, and therefore they are superior. And that right there is what eugenics is all about. People deserve to be treated with dignity and respect regardless of their health status. But healthism and BMI really push the binary idea that there is only one way to be healthy and acceptable by society's standards, and that is by being thin.

As I was writing this book, *The New York Times* published an article titled "Medical Group Says B.M.I. Alone Is Not Enough to Assess Health and Weight." Body mass index has long been used as the standard, but controversial, measurement of health. The American Medical Association is implementing a new policy that encourages doctors *not* to rely on BMI. The article opens with this statement:

> The American Medical Association voted to adopt a new pol-
> icy on Tuesday encouraging doctors not to rely only on body
> mass index, a long-used but potentially misleading metric,
> when assessing weight and health. The policy officially recog-
> nizes the "historical harm" of B.M.I. and states that the metric
> has been used "for racist exclusion."

Dr. Scott Hagan of the University of Washington, who wasn't involved with the decision to adopt the new policy, was quoted in the article as saying: "The B.M.I. is just a very poor measure of general health. . . . Someone with an elevated B.M.I. may be perfectly healthy." And yet, even though many healthcare professionals know this, they still pathologize their patients and cause harm by ignoring the nuances that affect people's health beyond their size.

One of these nuances is muscle mass, which BMI does not take into consideration, potentially leading someone who has a greater volume of muscle to be classified as "obese" or "overweight." In addition, your BMI does not tell your doctor about your access to food, or your ability to access safe or appropriate locations for movement, such as a walkable park and sidewalks.

When someone has a severe illness, such as cancer, that affects their health and potentially puts them at risk for premature death, having a higher BMI may in fact support a more favorable outcome during rigorous treatments such as therapies for cancer.[6]

On the flip side, however, is that someone with a higher BMI may still be malnourished. Eating disorders can happen to any person in any body, just as one's access to nutritious food will greatly impact their overall health regardless of BMI.

Public health campaigns often say that certain demographics° are at a higher risk for health conditions and that one way to improve your risk is to lower your BMI. This may be something you have experienced. People often ask me, "Well, if not reducing BMI, then what?" A client-centered provider should talk to you, their client. They should view you as a human being. They listen, they provide feedback. But they do not pathologize, they do not dictate. They help you make the best decision for you at that moment with what you have available. Because your gravitational pull on this Earth shouldn't be what determines how you are treated.

° When I was a community nutritionist, I began to notice that all the inner-city campaigns were aimed at reducing BMI. The materials included handouts briefly suggesting that it is easy to reduce your BMI by a few points. Remember, "reducing your BMI" is not a behavior. It is an outcome.

EL PROBLEMA WITH WEIGHT STIGMA

Weight stigma is weight-based discrimination, and it has a lot of implications for the health and well-being of those living in larger bodies. Ninety percent of my clients come to me after experiencing weight discrimination from healthcare providers, and the common thing I hear from them is despair.

Let's go back to Vanessa. I shared an overview of her history with doctors, but in this particular scenario, she went to see the doctor for a separate issue—her elbow was hurting. The doctor didn't even look at her or the elbow, or ask her any questions. Instead, they told her losing some weight would help her joints. Now, I know that you know that we *all* know an elbow is not a weight-bearing joint. It is heartbreaking and quite frankly ridiculous that a medical professional did not have the human decency to just look and speak to the person in front of them without biases coming up. Turns out my girl had tennis elbow from her repetitive duties at her job and her weight had nothing to do with it, but she had to go to a different doctor to get that diagnosis.

This assumption that the doctor made is a clear example of implicit bias. There are two types of bias that we can run into, especially within the healthcare community.

Implicit (unconscious) bias: This is a belief or stereotype that we hold unconsciously, without even realizing it. Implicit biases can be formed by experiences we have and our cultural backgrounds. We can have implicit biases based on race, age, weight, and gender and not realize how they affect our behaviors. Some examples include judging body health based on size, such as assuming someone in a larger body has diabetes, and believing that a white doctor knows more than a doctor who looks like your community members.

Explicit (conscious) bias:[7] This is a belief or stereotype that we hold consciously, that we are aware that we believe. People may choose to act on an explicit bias out of fear or defensiveness. You may have experienced explicit bias if you've been denied a job because of your race or hairstyle. Think about Vanessa's story: She was not given fair treatment for her condition because her doctor consciously chose to hone in on her body size instead.

BOTH TYPES OF bias can lead to poorer health outcomes for patients. It's important for healthcare professionals to acknowledge and address these biases to ensure equitable care for all patients.

In a paper published in the *International Journal of Obesity* in 2001,[8] the authors reported that doctors perceived their patients in larger bodies (or, as they state it, those with "obesity") as being more annoying, being noncompliant with treatment, and having worse self-control. Yup, you read that right. They labeled their patients "annoying," which is so ridiculous.

A study from 2012[9] revealed that the way a doctor chooses to address weight loss, if at all, is related to the BMI of the physician. That is, a normal-BMI doctor is more likely to address weight loss and BMI in patients if those patients are also a normal BMI or larger BMI than the doctor. On the other hand, a doctor with an overweight or obese BMI is less likely to engage in conversations about BMI or weight loss with patients. And in 2009,[10] in the journal *BMC Health Services Research,* researchers found that doctors showed less respect for patients with higher BMIs, demonstrating a conscious bias.

So what we are seeing here is that, regardless of someone's actual health, before the medical provider even sees their lab work, overweight patients are being judged. They are being labeled as lazy, annoying, and lacking willpower, which is complete bullshit.

The fight shouldn't be against "obesity," it should be against weight stigma. When there's a deeply embedded weight stigma in a healthcare system, patients don't get the care they need. This weight stigma leads to poor-quality healthcare and a greater incidence of chronic conditions.

Let's break down why weight stigma is so harmful.

Physical Implications

Lower quality of care: The three studies mentioned above demonstrated that misdiagnosis can occur when health issues are attributed to weight instead of looking for other causes and doing more lab work and medical tests.

Avoidance of healthcare: People are afraid of being judged for being in a bigger body (and for good reason!), so they avoid going for routine checkups, which may lead to conditions like high blood sugar, high cholesterol, high blood pressure, and even cancer being missed. Then, by the time they do go to the doctor, those conditions are out of control. If they had gone earlier, their conditions could have been monitored, nutritional modifications could have been started, and the disease might not have developed.

Weight cycling: This is repeated weight loss and gain, and for many people, part of the problem is feeling pressure to lose weight before they go to the doctor. This cycle can negatively impact metabolic health, leading to higher rates of heart disease, diabetes, and mortality.

Mental Health Implications

Mental distress: Weight stigma is associated with a 32 percent increase of depression in people compared to those who are in what is considered a normal-weight body, as well as a decrease in self-esteem.[11]

Preoccupation with food: Weight stigma leads to restriction in order to lose weight, which in turn may lead to a fixation on food because the person is hungry, and that can increase their risk for eating disorders.

Body dissatisfaction: Dissatisfaction with the body can lead someone to go to extremes to change it, increasing the risk for eating disorders.

These issues don't arise in just the medical system. Weight stigma occurs in all parts of life for those living in bigger bodies. Fat bodies* are discriminated against every day. Being told that, simply by existing, you are annoying or lazy will mess with anyone and can lead to disordered eating.

HOW DID WE GET HERE?

It's important to understand that diet culture and the way we view ourselves are rooted in the false idea that Eurocentric ways of eating are better. Let's go back to the idea of eugenics, and how its followers believed that the individual had full control over their health and how this made whites morally superior.

* I will use the term "fat" throughout the book, and you may hear people use the word "fat" to describe their body in a nonoffensive, neutral way. The thinking of fat liberationists encourages us to take the stigma out of the word.

Now you might be thinking, *How the heck is this tied to diet culture?* Well, it *really* is one and the same. We can trace thinness as the beauty ideal back to early American colonization and imperialism. In her book *Fearing the Black Body: The Racial Origins of Fat Phobia*,[12] Sabrina Strings, PhD, reveals that during the height of slavery, Europeans believed being thin and controlling what they ate made them morally superior. Therefore, they considered Black people to be inferior because of their bigger bodies.

In the late fifteenth century, as Europeans colonized other lands, they ventured into Africa and Asia, bringing with them a mix of disease and condescension. They often labeled Indigenous populations as "savages" and "gluttonous." In their quest for dominance, they imposed European religious beliefs, customs, and attire upon the Native peoples, reshaping centuries-old traditions. The echoes of these impositions are still palpable today, influencing everything from religious practices to fashion trends.

Beginning in the early sixteenth century, the transatlantic slave trade intensified the mockery and dehumanization of Black bodies, transforming them from exotic curiosities into commodified subjects. This dehumanization, coupled with racial theories and the many pseudoscientific beliefs of the eighteenth and nineteenth centuries, enabled enslavers to justify the brutality of their trade and deeply embedded their racist perceptions. In 1749, French author Georges-Louis Leclerc[13] garnered a substantial amount of recognition for his work in natural history, which later influenced the work of Darwin. In one chapter of Leclerc's well-known *Histoire naturelle, Générale et particulière*, he emphasized skin color as a primary difference among humans and then ranked body size and shape as secondary distinguishing features. He stereotypically described Black Africans as tall and well-built but naive and unintelligent. This echoed the biased views of earlier English intellectuals who associated being overweight with sluggishness and a lack of intelligence, and the rhetoric would be commonly accepted by society for centuries to come.

You see a lot of this anti-fat and racist rhetoric in women's magazines of the nineteenth century. In 1867, Mary Louise Booth signed on as the first editor of *Harper's Bazar* (as it was then spelled), which featured a series titled "For the Ugly Girls" that advised women on dietary habits. In volume five, forty-eighth edition, Susan Dunning Power answers a question from a reader who is lamenting her facial hair. Not only is it named ugly, but it's also tied back to food:

> These unfortunate cases are the result of morbid constitution, freaks of nature which are to be combated as one would eradicate leprosy or scrofula. The extreme growth of hair where it should not be comes from gross living, or in young persons is inherited from those whose blood is made of too rich materials.
>
> Living for two or three generations on overlarded meats, plenty of nice pastry, salt meats, ham, and fish, with good old pickles from brine—in short, what would be called high living among middle-class people—is pretty sure to leave its reminders on lip and brow.[14]

An article from 1877 titled "Our Women Growing Plump" emphasized that the slender physique of U.S. Anglo-Saxon females was more desirable than that of their European counterparts, mirroring sentiments from *Godey's Lady's Book*, a magazine dedicated to instructing women in the etiquette of white, Christian society.[15] Founded in 1830 as *The Lady's Book*, under its editor, Sarah Josepha Buell Hale, it emphasized women's moral growth, proper behavior in God's eyes, and moderation in consumption, and overeating was often associated with immorality and loss of beauty. In her book *Traits of American Life,* Hale offers the reminder:

> Eating to excess constantly will deaden or destroy the energies of the mind, while those of the animal are increased, till the immortal becomes perfectly swinish; and yet many tender, delicate mothers, seem to think that to make their children *eat,* is all that is requisite to make them *great.*[16]

Sabrina Strings's work is essential reading for developing an understanding of the origins of anti-fatness. We've already discussed that much explicit and implicit bias on weight comes from the medical field, but Strings's work identifies incidents even before those of the medical community. In her book *Fearing the Black Body,* Strings writes, "Racial scientific literature since at least the eighteenth century has claimed that fatness was 'savage' and 'black.'"[17]

This can be seen especially in the declared association between thinness and health in the Protestant community. Two names that were very prominent in the community were Sylvester Graham[18] (yes, of the graham cracker) and Dr. John Harvey Kellogg[19] (yes, of the cereal empire). Both men believed that eating a bland (no spices or spicy flavors) vegetarian diet, with lots of whole grains, vegetables, and fruits, would not only stop you from having inappropriate sexual thoughts and masturbating,* it would also improve your health and ensure moral virtue.

Kellogg led the eugenics movement in the United States and

---

* Cornflakes were invented as an anti-masturbation food, and if I have to know this, you need to know this because I will never stop laughing at it.

believed in creating a "new human race" by eating better and out-breeding the "savages." He encouraged white women to follow these diets, stay thin, and have a ton of babies because he basically believed the savages would die off. In his 1883 publication *Ladies' Guide in Health and Disease*, Kellogg argued that reforming women, who he deemed mentally inferior to men, could strengthen the American population, and claims that the reason Native Americans no longer occupied American lands was because earlier generations had "degenerated" due to poor health. (Note: He doesn't mention colonization.) He emphasized the link between a woman's diet, physique, and the overall health of the race. Kellogg was influential in merging medical perspectives with notions of ideal diet and weight for Americans, which magazines of the time, such as *Cosmopolitan,* promoted in their pages to the masses.

Although many of Dr. Kellogg's assertions were not born of medical science itself, he was considered a big shot in the medical community. Unfortunately some of his beliefs are still in medical books used now, and we can certainly see how his views linger in today's society.

THE MEDIA'S OBSESSION WITH THINNESS

We've seen how this conditioning toward the preferability of whiteness and thinness has persisted over the centuries and continues to damage individuals' feelings about not conforming to a certain type. Nowadays, this damage is often done through the media. In 2004, Anne E. Becker, PhD, MD,[20] conducted a landmark study on eating disorders in young women in the island nation of Fiji. There were two phases. Part one, in 1995, occurred just after television service was introduced in a rural community in Fiji, and phase two took place in 1998, when girls in secondary school were interviewed. The study found:

1. In 1995, only a few of the girls reported dieting to lose weight, and none reported self-induced vomiting. Most girls reported relatively high body satisfaction.
2. In 1998, the study found significant changes. Nearly three-quarters of the girls reported feeling "too big" or fat at least sometimes. Dieting was reported by 69 percent of the girls, and self-induced vomiting to control weight was reported by 11.3 percent.
3. The study also found that girls who lived in a house with a television were more than three times as likely to have attitudes and behaviors indicative of an eating disorder.

This might be Fiji, but we can see that this translates all around the world, especially in the United States. You might not know that in Latin America, American television programming was the main source of entertainment media in the 1980s and '90s. We watched popular American shows dubbed in Spanish or we watched telenovelas, which heavily emphasized Eurocentric beauty ideals. Our culture's current obsession with thinness is very steeped in acculturation, which is the process of adopting a new culture. In this case, as Latines living in the United States, we often feel pressured to conform to Western beauty ideals so we can fit in. And these beauty ideals almost always prioritize thinness.

American TV shows like *Friends* and *Baywatch,* both of which were popular in Latin America, presented a narrow, Western beauty ideal that emphasized slender, white, and blond bodies. For many of us, consistent exposure to these images leads to feelings of inadequacy and pressure to conform. Additionally, the

American lifestyle and culture portrayed pushed viewers toward Americanization, which sometimes is at odds with our own traditions. This blend of entertainment and subtle cultural imposition influenced both individuals' body image and broader cultural perceptions.

Also, fat bodies are generally described in literature and depicted in movies in derogatory terms, and these narratives teach us that a character is not lovable until they are skinny and pretty, that they do not matter until they lose weight, that no matter how hard they try, it is not until they are skinny that they are seen. Just think of the character Monica in *Friends* or Schmidt in *New Girl*.

It is mind-boggling how these shows perpetuated what beauty should be. Just the other day, I saw *Baywatch* come on TV and thought to myself, *Holy shit, these women were THIN*. And no, I am not shaming them. It was the 1990s and we all know that "thin thin" was in then, when heroin chic was considered the ideal.

Many of us grew up in an era when extreme thinness was praised and considered the peak of health and beauty. In a *New York Times* article titled "A Death Tarnishes Fashion's 'Heroin Look,'"[21] the author states:

> After years of denial by the fashion industry that heroin use among its players had any relation to the so-called heroin-chic style of fashion photography that has become so prevalent, the fatal overdose of Davide Sorrenti, 20, a promising photographer at the heart of the scene, was like a small bomb going off.

Even though the idea of "heroin chic" eventually faded away as people came to terms with how unhealthy it was, it still became a staple among many young women growing up in the '90s. We were bombarded with pictures of supermodels like Kate Moss and Naomi Campbell taken by photographers looking to connect popular culture (such as Kurt Cobain, drug use among models, the '90s party scene) to fashion. Because of this approach to fashion advertising, we began to associate thinness with health and beauty.

Latine communities have often been underrepresented in the media (unless it's the Miss Universe pageant), and that lack of culturally appropriate content, in addition to selling us this "ideal look," also sold us the American Dream via these shows and fashion. Whether we want to come to terms with it or not, the American Dream included—and still does—being thin, white, blond, and preferably running down a beach in a red bikini like Pamela Anderson or, even better for our teenage selves, looking like the twins from Sweet Valley High (woo, did those books have a chokehold on me). We were seriously left thinking that there was only one way to look in order to fit in. You don't need a doctor to tell you your BMI to want to lose weight, because the pressure is everywhere.

When we consider all the different ways we've been conditioned to value thinness, it's no wonder disordered eating and eating disorders are on the rise. Between 2000 and 2018, the prevalence of eating disorders worldwide more than doubled.[22]

Eating Disorders and Disordered Eating

Eating disorders are a mental health issue. Rates of binge eating disorder and bulimia, the most prevalent of the disorders in the Latine community, are on the rise. Unfortunately, these illnesses go undetected and undiagnosed in our communities mostly due to racism. BIPOC individuals are far less likely to be diagnosed with eating disorders than their white counterparts, even though rates of these disorders are comparable. This underdiagnosis doesn't just delay treatment, it also contributes to the $64.7 billion annual economic burden of eating disorders in the United States.[23] These disparities hit underserved communities the hardest, where access to culturally competent care is already limited, deepening existing healthcare inequalities.[24]

Eating disorders are mental health conditions under criteria set out in the *DSM-5*, the *Diagnostic and Statistical Manual of Mental Disorders, Fifth Edition,* and they require clinical intervention due to the significant mental and physical health risks they pose. Eating disorders included in the *DSM-5* include anorexia, bulimia, and binge eating.

Disordered eating is a range of irregular eating behaviors that may or may not warrant diagnosis. Examples include chronic yo-yo dieting, having feelings of guilt and shame related to eating, frequent weight fluctuation, adhering to rigid rules and routines concerning food (as with orthorexia nervosa, an obsession with eating healthy), and preoccupation with food, body size, and weight. In an online survey by *Carolina Public Health* and *SELF* magazine,[25] 75 percent of women in the United States reported disordered eating behaviors and 53 percent of dieters were already at a healthy weight but still wanted to lose more.

I don't know about you, but this describes about 90 percent of the women in my personal and professional life. A study published in *JAMA Pediatrics* reports that one out of five adolescents has a disordered eating pattern, with an increased risk for girls compared to boys.[26]

Children and teenagers need calories, aka energy, to grow. While calories are our body's energy source, today the concept of calories is unfortunately tied to restriction and changing the body's appearance. Puberty and adolescence are years of rapid growth, with bone generation being so fast that growth spurts seem to happen overnight. Calorie restriction and dieting only hurt children. It is important for them to eat adequately, consistently, and with variety.

Eating Disorders in the Latine Community

Eating disorders affect people in all types of bodies and of all races and ethnicities. But unfortunately, the face of eating disorders is the thin, frail white woman. We see it in ads, and we see it on television and in other media. I particularly think of the 2017 Netflix movie *To the Bone,* which starred Lily Collins and Keanu Reeves. We even see it when looking at brochures for eating disorder treatment centers.

While we know that eating disorders are an issue in this country, with 9 percent of the population experiencing one at some point in their lifetime,[27] unfortunately, in the Latine community, this number is grossly underreported. We don't often think of eating disorders as having an effect on us, and this can lead to healthcare practitioners missing key signs that something is wrong.

COMMUNITY STIGMA AROUND EATING DISORDERS

I also think one of the reasons we don't really talk about eating disorders in our community is because the phrase for it feels weird in Spanish: trastorno de alimentación. In my Dominican way of speaking that sounds a little bougie, I can see the tías going, "Que trastorno ni que trastorno. Coño, usted come y ya!"

Because why would we feel this way about eating? We are given food and we should be grateful for it, right? Think about it: For our communities, when we are given anything, we should accept it without question and be filled with gratitude. We are in this country of so-called opportunity, and we are being fed and have a roof over our heads, and according to them, we are much better off than those going hungry in places all over the world that they can list. This is true, but two truths can always coexist.

Yes, we have access to food, but we are also immersed in a world that values thinness, and everywhere you look—on social media, in the medical system, in many aspects of life—everyone is in pursuit of thinness, which grants us proximity to whiteness, and that whiteness allows us to be finally seen and heard. And who doesn't want to be seen and heard?

However, the effects of the denial of mental health issues and eating disorders as well as colonization within our communities have contributed to the challenge of comprehending mental health issues and trauma whether we acknowledge it or not. As many elders in our communities have often emphasized, they didn't have the luxury of acknowledging feelings of depression or anxiety. This sentiment is often echoed in households like mine, where discussing our emotional struggles was not the norm. When I mention attending therapy, my father's favorite response is "Usted no está loca, no necesitas terapia."

We are conditioned not to openly express our emotional concerns, and this is passed down through generations. My inability to suppress my emotions earned me the label "dramatica" because I refuse to bottle up my feelings—your girl is a crier. However, we need to be able to acknowledge that our upbringing and its prohibition of addressing our emotions and well-being has only left us grappling with said feelings and dealing with many mental health issues.

I found a few studies[28, 29, 30] that show the significance of acculturation and intergenerational conflict within the Latine community, and how they combine with our tendencies to suppress emotions to shape our perceptions of mental health and emotional struggles. However, another critical aspect of overall well-being also contributes to the challenges we face: food scarcity or insecurity.

Research indicates that food scarcity (the total amount of food available to a population) and food insecurity (one's ability to access food)[31] are pervasive concerns within the Latine community, particularly among immigrants and low-income families. The interplay between acculturation and these food-related challenges can lead to higher incidences of eating disorders. In my experience as a dietitian, people who have had less access to food growing up can develop behaviors such as fear of underbuying food, overeating out of fear of not having enough, and ignoring body cues for hunger or fullness due to their relationship with food waste. Research on this topic indicates that Latinos, especially those born in the United States or who spent a larger percentage of their life in the United States, are at greater risk for eating disorders such as binge eating and bulimia. This risk also correlates with low levels of education, which we will address along with social determinants of health in Chapter 6.[32] Acculturation often involves the adoption of Western diets and eating habits, which may add to concerns related to body image and weight. This can contribute to the onset of eating disorders, especially as one navigates the expectation to be thin and "American enough."

One relevant study, titled "Epidemiology of Eating Disorders in Latin America," addresses the prevalence of eating disorders in the Latin American region.[33] Additionally, the study "Understanding Eating Disorders Among Latinas"[34] has been instrumental in deepening awareness of eating disorders specifically among Latina individuals.

To break this cycle, it is crucial to foster open conversations about mental health and emotional struggles within our communities, and to acknowledge that mental health is a valid concern that deserves attention. Addressing food scarcity and insecurity, while also promoting healthy habits that respect diverse cultural backgrounds, can help mitigate the risk factors associated with eating disorders.

The first step in providing support is removing stigma. Just the other day, my mom was watching some Spanish TV show and a person was discussing the power of positive thinking and how medication should not be used for anxiety because we can just think away the issues by being positive. Look, there are times when, yes, we can think positively and feel better, but anxiety, depression, eating disorders, and other mental health issues cannot simply be cured by buenas vibras. Toxic positivity—an attitude that we should suppress all bad feelings—can be so instilled in us and our culture that we don't recognize the issues right in front of us because we refuse to acknowledge them. Some people need therapy and medication, and there should be *zero* shame in asking for and getting help. It really warms my heart that so many of us are breaking these generational strictures to be better for ourselves and the generations after us.

The more that we interrogate these unhealthy patterns that have been perpetuated in our media and communities for years, the better equipped we will be to dismantle diet culture and prevent it from leaking into various facets of our lives. Then we can face them head-on.

Let's go back to Vanessa. It took many months of working together to undo a lot of the fears she had related to our foods that were instilled in her not just by her doctor, but also by the conditioning she was given at a young age. We had to break down her fears and focus on her actual health by discussing in depth the nutritional content of our cultural foods and learning about what constitutes a complete meal and how to disconnect weight from health. Although that can all be scary, it can also be very liberating. Ultimately, Vanessa was able to let go of her obsession with weight and find a doctor who saw past the numbers. She was able to find health on her own terms, nourish her body, and work out in a way that led her to feeling better and having amazing lab work.

TLDR: The obsession with being thin leads to disordered eating and eating disorders. This desire comes from wanting to be healthy, but also to meet societal pressures to conform to the thin ideal. In the Latino community, and especially for first-gen Americans, we are dealing with acculturation and fitting in. The thin ideal is rooted in white supremacy and eugenics, which have infiltrated the medical system in the use of BMI and increased the prevalence of weight stigma. BMI is not a great indicator of health, and overemphasizing it can lead to weight stigma and poorer health outcomes. Disordered eating, which affects so many people, is often mistaken for healthy eating habits. Our body image is fucked because we have been taught that thinness and European features are ideal, and that is not true.

CHULA PRACTICE: Check out the following texts to deepen your understanding of the topics discussed in this chapter:

Sabrina Strings, *Fearing the Black Body*

Sonya Renee Taylor, *The Body Is Not an Apology*

Roxane Gay, *Hunger*

Da'Shaun L. Harrison, *Belly of the Beast*

Chrissy King, *The Body Liberation Project*

Mikki Kendall, *Hood Feminism*

2

WHY IS DIET CULTURE
STILL AROUND?

Chula Story: Yocayra

YOCAYRA is thirty-two. Her mother was diagnosed with type 2 diabetes at the age of fifty, and it sent her whole family on a health journey. Yocayra felt she had to "fix" her health ASAP if she wanted a different outcome. With the help of an online community, she began her keto journey. After three months of an on-and-off relationship with the keto diet, she found herself at her annual checkup and much to her surprise, her cholesterol level had risen by more than a hundred points. The doctor handed her a sheet of paper describing a low-carb diet in terms of the U.S. Department of Agriculture's MyPlate, which sets out what proportion of each food group you should eat for a balanced diet. The one MyPlate example that stood out to her was brown rice, broccoli, and grilled chicken. She was distraught and vowed not to go on any fad diets. She was going to work on her health via lifestyle. She wanted to make sure she focused on clean eating by eating real and whole foods like her ancestors ate.

She didn't intend to lose weight, but her doctor had suggested that losing five to ten pounds would help bring down her choles-terol. Yocayra had never focused on weight loss, but she thought, *How hard can it be?*

She started following me online a few months after she began her journey. Finding a dietitian who looked like her was very important to her. But after a few weeks of following me, she started questioning her health journey. Were the new lifestyle rules she'd started to follow *actually* helping? Or was she just stressing herself the fuck out?

Yocayra's experience is a great example of how diets remain relevant in our day-to-day lives, even when we might not be actively seeking them out.

Let's take a moment to discuss intentional weight loss, which is what diets and many lifestyle changes sell. This is the intentional restriction of foods to lose weight, which means that you are more than likely restricting calories, micromanaging food, and over-exercising. Those are not healthy, sustainable behaviors. I know damn well that you know that having to count every calorie every day is not fun, and when your weight plateaus, it only leads to more restriction, and the mental Olympics never stop. But if that's how you want to live, you have that bodily autonomy.

We, however, have evidence that this does not work. The Minnesota Starvation Experiment[1] is a prime example of how intentional weight loss can lead us on a slippery slope into diet culture and disordered eating. The results are so wild, you will never unsee it.

MINNESOTA STARVATION EXPERIMENT

The Minnesota Starvation Experiment[2] was a landmark study conducted during World War II to understand the physical and psychological effects of severe food restriction and to determine the best way to safely reintroduce food to extremely malnourished people to avoid the severe metabolic effects that "refeeding" can cause. Conducted by Ancel Keys, the same guy who studied BMI, the Minnesota Starvation Experiment may seem similar to diet blogs and weight-loss programs you've seen in the present day that promote weeks of intentional calorie restriction. Keys's goal was to guide public health interventions to help concentration camp victims and the emaciated citizens of German-occupied Europe recover from extreme food deprivation. What he did not know was that his study would later be used in eating disorder research.

Keys recruited thirty-six healthy men who did not go to war for religious or moral reasons, and they underwent extensive medical and psychological evaluations to ensure that they were in good health. They were between the ages of twenty-two and thirty-three, and from various educational and occupational backgrounds. Each had to walk or run twenty-two miles per week to simulate the physical exertion of someone in a famine. During the experiment's first phase, a period of twelve weeks, they were fed 3,200 calories per day and monitored for behavior, health, and energy in order to establish baseline data. The semistarvation phase lasted twenty-four weeks, when they were given a 1,570-calorie diet*—half of what they had been eating.

The men were then placed in a twelve-week restricted rehabilitation phase during which they were fed 2,000 to 3,000 calories a day to study the effects of refeeding. This was followed by eight weeks of unrestricted rehab, during which they were allowed to eat as much as they wanted to so as to regain weight and recover.

---

* How many of you have been encouraged to reduce your intake to this calorie amount or lower by a trainer, influencer, healthcare professional, or magazine, suggesting that it is enough food?

Throughout each phase, the study participants were observed for behavioral and bodily changes. To put it briefly, the men experienced intense symptoms, and shit got weird.

Physical Changes

After the semistarvation phase, participants had lost 25 percent of their initial weight and had substantial decreases in strength, endurance, temperature, and heart rate. There was a significant reduction in their heart size and a 10 percent decrease of heart blood volume. They also lost a dramatic amount of muscle mass.

Changes in reproductive function were also reported, with lower sex drive identified among the participants. Although specifics on sperm count were not reported, we know that extreme calorie deficits and weight loss can lead to hormonal imbalances that reduce sex drive and more. So when the girlies are selling you restriction to balance your hormones, think twice.

Psychological Changes

Depression, irritability, and moodiness increased significantly throughout the semistarvation phase. Attention span declined, and there was a noticeable increase in the incidence of neurotic behaviors such as an obsession with food and collecting cookbooks and recipes. (At the time of this writing, I observe another form of "neurotic behavior" presented to us in the form of relentless social media reminders of super-high-protein meals, "What I Eat in A Day" videos, and body checking—that is, showing how your body has changed in your reflection of your camera.)

Social and Emotional Impact

The men in the experiment became withdrawn and avoided interaction with others. During the semistarvation phase, the participants reported feelings of intense hunger, fatigue, and apathy. Gum chewing became prevalent as a way to keep the mouth occupied in the face of constant hunger. Some men were reported to chew up to forty packs of gum a day, and because of the high demand, Keys had to limit the amount they could chew. Participants in this experiment reportedly became so distraught that they broke dietary rules by eating scraps of food from garbage cans and stealing food. One participant was removed from the experiment due to his behavior impeding his ability to follow the restrictive diet.

Cognitive Effects

The men's cognition was impaired, with declines in concentration and comprehension as well as judgment reported during and following the semistarvation phase.

Long-Term Consequences

Even after the refeeding phase, a preoccupation with food persisted and the men faced many struggles with disordered eating behaviors. Despite returning to their regular diets, they felt an extreme sense of hunger and consistently overate. After the study, it took years for them to recover from the physiological and mental health issues that they experienced.

Does any of what these men went through feel familiar? Because if I am being honest, it's what 99 percent of the women I work with experience. And the experiment's restrictions are what I see day in and day out on the internet being promoted by mommy bloggers, vloggers, dietitians, and influencers. A lot of disordered-eating issues are chalked up to the person having no willpower or needing to restrict more and be better. But the truth is, the more you restrict, the more issues arise and become harder to ignore. These men were only semistarved, and women today semistarve themselves in the name of health and diets every other month in a vicious cycle that only leads to more stress. In a modern world where most have adequate access to food, how is it possible that we purposely starve ourselves in the name of health?

DIET CULTURE DOESN'T GET TO STEAL HEALTHY BEHAVIORS

Let's talk about healthy behaviors. Healthy behaviors are different elements of your life that positively shape your overall health. I consider them what happens when you just live; they're not meant to stress you out, but the truth is that diet culture can take healthy behaviors to the extreme, and that can become stressful. Here is how I like to think about healthy behaviors and the good and the bad:

Health Element	What Restriction Teaches Us	Authentic Health con sazón Latina
Sleep	Getting less sleep equals more productivity. Prioritize work over rest.	Sleep is crucial for overall well-being, allowing time for essential functions like cell repair and hormone regulation. Prioritize descanso. Taking time to rest is an act of self-care; it's a rebellion against hustle culture. You deserve it—you do not need to earn it.

Health Element	What Restriction Teaches Us	Authentic Health con sazón Latina
Nutrition	Restrict foods. Count calories. Obsess over macronutrients, especially protein.	Eating is the ultimate act of self-care. Explore nutrient-rich Latine foods. Learn to add nutrition by adding ingredients and dishes to meals.
Exercise	More is better. Take no days off. Adhere to extreme routines.	Movimiento is about balance and listening to your cuerpo. Dance, take a walk, throw some tires—choose what feels good to you. Make an exercise routine that is a part of your life, not your whole life. Leave time for rest and recovery, and allow yourself modifications and flexibility.
Stress Management	Prioritize hustle over health. Don't take breaks.	Properly manage stress. Latines are at higher risk for developing diabetes and heart disease, both of which can be influenced by stress, so making its management a priority is key. Take breaks, and prioritize joy.
Meal Prep	Stick to strict menus of monotonous foods in calorie-driven plans.	Meal prepping does not have to be hard. I like framing it as "menu creation," not "meal planning." Involve the family, pick themes, take advantage of leftovers and takeout. Lean on convenience. Menu creation should reduce stress, not cause it.

Health Element	What Restriction Teaches Us	Authentic Health con sazón Latina
Salads and Veggies	Eat only bland, low-calorie options that are "good" and virtuous rather than higher-calorie meals.	Salads and veggies don't have to be bland and flavorless or boring—think ensaladas with avocado, lime, and grilled corn. And use salad dressings, which contain fats that are essential for nutrient absorption.
Diet Foods	Allow yourself only guilt-free, low-calorie versions of "bad" foods.	If you like a diet soda, that is perfectly fine. The key is intention: Don't eat or drink something because it's labeled "better"; you should genuinely like it. Also, remember that low-calorie foods are low-energy foods.

THE DIETS WE ALL KNOW (AND STRESS OVER)

Diet culture takes eating to the extreme, to a point where you're more stressed than actually enjoying life. When I say "Diet culture doesn't get to steal healthy behaviors," I mean that you can do these healthy behaviors in a way that doesn't stress you out. I remind my clients to make small shifts (I call them 1 percent lifts) that add up over time to bring habitual change, such as making sure you precut your veggies and fruits (or buy them precut) so they're easily available during the week.

My approach is not sexy. It isn't going to help you lose ten pounds in ten days. We are drawn to diets because they present a clear plan, straightforward rules, and an opportunity to be in control of a "problem" (aka your body) that needs to be "solved."

Diets come and go over the decades, and new ones continue to make their way into the wellness space as the latest "gold standard" diet. Even though some diets are now recognized as being bad for us, diets have a way of reinventing themselves and adapting to the current moment in order to seem like weight loss is more "attainable" and the restrictions prescribed are less problematic. It's not uncommon for a diet like Atkins to come back as the slightly different keto. They're almost as trendy as fashion.

Low-Fat Diets

The low-fat diet was super popular in the 1990s, and some of my older clients still follow it. Essentially, fat is a no-no, a restriction stemming from the fear of becoming fat. The NIH—National Institutes of Health—defines a food as "low fat" if it has three grams or less of fat per serving.

In the 1990s, we saw an explosion of low-fat products on the shelves of grocery stores. People were baking everything with as little fat as possible, using canned spray oils, getting their salad dressing on the side and dipping each individual piece of lettuce into the little cup it came in. Let me clarify: Doing any of this is not inherently bad; it's the intention and the accompanying shame that cause the issue. It stems from the idea that eating fat will make you fat and give you heart disease. We know that is not true—one single food or ingredient can't cause a disease. But in the '90s, so many people believed this. Thankfully, this idea that fat is the source of heart issues has been debunked. In fact, adding plant fats such as those in nuts, seeds, and oils can help with cholesterol. Eventually this diet trend changed, and the pendulum swung to the opposite side and now we have the "keto" (ketogenic) diet because when you have less fat, you have more carbs.

HIGH-FAT, LOW-CARB DIETS

The keto diet is a high-fat diet that only allows you twenty to fifty grams of carbohydrates a day. Before we go any further, let me make something clear: YOUR BRAIN'S PREFERRED SOURCE OF ENERGY IS GLUCOSE, WHICH YOUR BODY MAKES BY BREAKING DOWN CARBOHYDRATES!

Stans of the keto diet will argue that the brain will use ketones instead of glucose, which is true, but just because the brain can use its plan B option doesn't make it healthy. Glucose is our preferred source of energy, and by burning it is how the brain functions the best. And just to be completely clear here: If you made the choice to do keto and you liked it and it worked for you, do not message me and tell me that. I love that for you, but this message is for those who tried it, realized it was not sustainable, and are looking for a different way. You do you, boo.

It's a little-known fact that the keto diet was originally designed to be used in epilepsy treatment, but because lowering the amount of carbs in your diet does burn more fat, it became popular as a weight-loss diet. But just because it's popular doesn't mean it's healthy. Here are a few reasons I don't recommend keto:

1. Nutrient deficiencies: Restricting carbs can lead to inadequate intake of essential nutrients like vitamins, minerals, and fiber.
2. "Keto flu": Transitioning into ketosis can cause temporary symptoms like fatigue, headaches, irritability, nausea, and constipation, which do not sound fun, and I don't understand why anyone would put themselves through this.
3. Increased saturated fat intake: The keto diet may lead to consuming a high amount of saturated fats, which can impact heart health.

4. Potential for muscle loss: Low glucose availability while on keto may result in muscle loss because the body can also use protein from its own muscles to produce glucose with inadequate carbohydrate intake. Because people tend to eat a substantial amount of protein when going "keto" or low carb, their body does not enter a ketotic state. Instead, the body breaks down its own protein for glucose first. The true ketogenic diet approach is low to moderate, not high, protein intake for this reason. However, this is not something you see on social media!

5. Limited food choices and adherence: The strict carb restriction of keto can make it hard to stick to the diet in the long term and isolates you from social gatherings, which can in turn affect your mental health.

Let's revisit Yocayra, who went into the keto diet filled with hope to reduce her carb intake so she could prevent the same diagnosis her mom had recently received. What she did not realize was that her low consumption of fiber paired with the high intake of saturated fats would increase her cholesterol levels. And not only that, eating low carb can also cause the muscle loss I mentioned above because we have a nifty mechanism called gluconeogenesis, which is the process by which protein is broken down into glucose when we are not eating enough carbohydrates for energy. This protein comes from our own muscles and from what we eat. Essentially, you are eating yourself from the inside out! With less muscle tissue, over time, we have fewer insulin receptors, which are needed to metabolize glucose, and this can lead to insulin resistance. Insulin is the hormonal key that allows glucose into the cell for burning, and where there is insulin resistance, the cell won't accept the key, leading to high blood sugar and, in turn, a higher risk for diabetes. Essentially, the diet Yocayra thought would help prevent diabetes could possibly cause it.

Raw Food Diets

Raw food diets are all about consuming predominantly uncooked and unprocessed foods. Proponents assert that heating foods can destroy certain nutrients and natural enzymes. While some vitamins, such as vitamin C, are sensitive to heat, cooking can enhance the availability of compounds like lycopene in tomatoes and beta-carotene in carrots. These diets typically consist of fruits, vegetables, nuts, seeds, and sometimes sprouted grains and legumes.

Of course, none of this is bad, but again, the intention behind it and how it makes you feel are key. I understand why someone would try this—you're just eating foods that are healthy. I encourage this; however, the rigidity of the restrictions is a problem. I want you to be able to eat arroz con habichuelas and not have an anxiety attack over it having been cooked. Cooking some foods allows more nutrition to come through, and it adds flavor and texture.[3] Sticking to rules like only eating raw foods only adds stress, and in the long run, you get burned out from not being able to enjoy all the foods you love, which ultimately backfires.

Meal Replacement Shakes / Very Low-Calorie Diets

And then there are the three-shakes-a-day, super-low-calorie diets that restrict you the most. I will not name the company that promotes this and preys on the Latino community because they are my arch nemesis and I do not speak their name. But the chokehold that these shakes have on people is wild. They are loaded with low-calorie sweeteners (nothing wrong with them) and fiber to make you feel super full and give you the illusion of having eaten enough.

Now, I get it. Having a shake is so easy, you don't have to think. It gives you a sense of control. You are able to just blend a powder with water and *boom,* a meal. The issue is that these are too low-calorie, filling you up with fiber and liquid to mask the hunger and give you a false sense of fullness. But it's not sustainable, and eventually, the hunger will kick in, possibly leading to the binge-restrict cycle.

IT'S A LIFESTYLE, NOT A DIET, DUH!

At this point, I know that you know diets are bad, duh. You do not diet! You, on the other hand, are just trying to live a healthy lifestyle. You may have heard the phrase "It's not a diet, it's a lifestyle." This is what I call dieting on the DL.

Yocayra technically was not on a diet; she was just trying to eat healthier. But in the process, she was following so many rules. If your lifestyle doesn't allow you to spontaneously eat your abuela's dessert (because it tastes good) and forces you to burn off the calories, it's not a lifestyle, it's a diet. As of 2024, if you check the "Healthy Lifestyle" hashtag on Instagram, you get almost 133 million posts. I also counted thirteen flexible-diet lifestyle books in a quick Google search. Flexible dieting is an eating style that suggests you still get to eat whatever you want but you have guidelines to follow, such as a high protein or vegetable intake goal. This is similar to the "80/20" mentality in which you follow your dietary rules 80 percent of the time, eating whatever you want for 20 percent.

Let's make the connection here. What is happening when folks see diets as bad? They run to take a "lifestyle" approach, but then it turns out that this "lifestyle" doesn't allow them to actually live a more flexible life at all. Instead, it's creating unnecessary stress.

Calories in Versus Calories Out

If you're on social media, it's nearly impossible to ignore the calories in, calories out (CICO) influencer posts. When someone is yelling "Calories in, calories out!" they are talking about the energy you eat and the energy you burn and how to find a balance of the two that will make you lose weight. The idea that weight management is solely a matter of calories in versus calories out oversimplifies the complex factors that influence our bodies and health. Our bodies are not simple math equations. They are smart and efficient systems influenced by genetics, hormones, metabolism, and even our unique microbiomes, and all of these play vital roles in how our bodies process and store energy. This means that the number of calories we eat and burn does not tell the whole story.

Our bodies are wired for survival. When we restrict our calorie intake or engage in excessive exercise, our metabolism adjusts to conserve energy. This can lead to a cycle of yo-yo dieting and weight regain, which can be frustrating and damaging to our overall well-being. Research supports the idea that weight regulation involves a complex interplay of various factors beyond simple calories. Elements such as genetics, hormones, stress, sleep, and psychological well-being all contribute to our body weight and shape. The focus should shift from rigid calorie counting to adopting a balanced and sustainable lifestyle that promotes overall health and well-being, like what I described in the Introduction. But instead, we have a medical system that 100 percent knows that restriction and yo-yo dieting are harmful to your health but still promotes it because of the fatphobia we have in this country.

If It Fits Your Macros

Macros, or macronutrients, are the three major components of our diet: protein, carbohydrates, and fats. While it's true that they play important roles in our nutrition, solely focusing on macros as a means to achieving health or weight goals can be a slippery slope. It is not uncommon to see social media posts that recommend a certain amount of macronutrients you need in a meal and "What I Eat in a Day" videos showing you how to hit a macronutrient goal such as eating a certain amount of protein. The If It Fits Your Macros approach promotes the idea that certain ratios or specific amounts of macros are the key to success, which can create an unhealthy obsession with numbers and rigid dietary rules. It's important to remember that our bodies are complex, and eating and nourishing the body goes beyond micromanaging food.

Having an awareness of macronutrients is not inherently a part of diet culture, but micromanaging your food intake by measuring grams can be a diet. In macro counting, protein becomes the "it girl," the Regina George, if you will. Typically, when someone is prescribed a macronutrient goal, it is based on a weight-loss goal and not someone's dietary preferences, such as if they are vegetarian or prefer more complex carbohydrates. This focus on nutrition may consider cultural foods such as beans to have too many carbs and avocados too much fat when in reality, these two foods are highly nourishing.

Tracking and crafting meals to "fit your macros" takes a lot of work because you need to divide your plate, weigh ingredients, and be perfect. Often a perfect dish looks like unseasoned chicken, brown rice, and broccoli, and we repeatedly make this dish because we know it fits our macros. This then takes away the ability to go to your abuela's house and eat the ropa vieja or the mangu she made. The biggest pitfall of the If It Fits Your Macros approach is that if you can't track it, you can't eat it.

However, food is not a monolith; most foods are composed of a few if not all the macros. That makes counting macros so tedious. Have you ever tried adding sancocho to MyFitnessPal? You can't, because we do not eat macronutrients separately, and we shouldn't! It just adds more stress that you do not need to your life.

Clean Eating and Unprocessed Foods

Yocayra decided to move to a clean eating approach because shouldn't natural, unprocessed foods be best? Isn't that the way our ancestors ate? But the thing about clean eating that we often forget is that it's about food morality and hierarchy.

The concept of clean eating suggests that some foods are inherently "clean" and others are "dirty," placing a moral value judgment on what we eat. But here's the truth: Food should not carry guilt or shame. Labeling certain foods as clean or dirty can lead to restrictive eating patterns, disordered relationships with food, and a distorted view of nutrition. It puts foods into buckets that stress you the hell out.

People assume organic foods are "clean" and healthy. According to the U.S. Department of Agriculture, "Produce can be called organic if it's certified to have grown on soil that had no prohibited substances applied for three years prior to harvest. Prohibited substances include most synthetic fertilizers and pesticides." "Organic" is solely about the method of production, not a nutritional label. I want you to understand that being labeled "organic" does not inherently increase the nutrition of a food. I see this a lot with my low-income clients who are so worried about eating clean after watching a documentary that suggested organic foods were the only way to become healthy. These clients aren't able to afford organic foods because they are more expensive than conventional produce, sometimes as high as 20 percent more.[4] All people should be able to eat, and despite what influencers are touting during their grocery hauls, conventionally grown nonorganic foods have nutritional value. But diet culture thrives on fearmongering and will continue to do so until we dismantle it.

I wish we focused our energy on identifying ways to support sustainable farms, local farmers, and ethical practices for farmworkers. Processed foods are often discussed but rarely understood in their full complexity, especially in the clean-eating world. Now, what do we mean when we say "processed foods"? When we say a food is processed, we're talking about it having undergone any method used to transform its raw ingredients into a more convenient, palatable, or shelf-stable form. This can be as simple as chopping up vegetables, or as complex as canning or fermenting. We've got mechanical processing, which includes physical changes like grinding wheat into flour. Thermal processing involves heat and includes methods like pasteurization and canning. Chemical processing might involve adding preservatives or other substances, and then there's fermentation, where microorganisms are used to alter the food. So, "processed" doesn't necessarily mean it's bad for you. There's a wide range of what processed food can be, from items like frozen peas to ultraprocessed foods like oatmilk.

I understand the desire to eat like our ancestors and eat fewer processed foods. It makes total sense: There was less processed food a hundred years ago. And people did not live as long as they do now and did not practice certain health-promoting behaviors such as handwashing. But there were also a lot of other fucked-up practices. In addition, capitalism and climate change have changed our access to food and our ability to grow, forage, and provide nutrition for ourselves and others. Going back to our roots is largely impossible due to the industrialization of food production. In so many ways we cannot eat like our ancestors did, but we can certainly get close to it and reclaim it.

We need to remove the shame and guilt that are often associated with relying on processed foods. We can use these foods to our advantage to help reduce stress. And we can always add nutrition to them. For instance, why not throw some canned beans and frozen vegetables into that instant rice? Or what about adding frozen fruits to oatmeal? Simple tweaks can make all the difference, adding fiber, vitamins, and other essential nutrients to your meals.

If you are working forty hours a week and trying to juggle life and social pressures, cooking and prepping time might not always be available, and leaning into convenience is key. Remember, capitalism and the structure of modern work often make processed foods a necessary choice, not a "lazy" or "unhealthy" one. So let's get rid of the judgment and recognize that people are doing the best they can within systems that often don't support us. Rather than pointing fingers, how about looking at ways to elevate these processed choices?

Let's shift the conversation away from guilt-tripping the individual and toward lessening the impact of systemic issues and coming up with practical solutions. Viewing things with a more balanced perspective can help us understand that "healthy eating" can look very different for each person based on their unique circumstances. By acknowledging the complexities and challenges people face, we not only remove shame but also empower everyone to make better-informed choices, no matter what their situation.

DIETS DON'T WORK, BUT THEY DO CAUSE DAMAGE

At this point, you have a pretty good idea of why diets do not work. Even though we may recognize their faults, I think most of us want diets to work because we want to be accepted. As a person who can walk through life being mostly accepted as thin, I will never truly know how it feels to be faced with that overwhelming pressure to make one's body conform to what's deemed "normal," which is why I will never—and I mean *never*—shame you for going on a diet, for wanting to lose weight, or for just wanting to fit in. Because the truth of the matter is, being thinner brings us closer to whiteness and closer to being seen, and at the end of the day, who doesn't want to be seen?

Diets can also help us feel in control. When so much in our lives feels out of control, diets give us a false sense of control over our bodies and our health, and because health and thinness are synonymous in our culture, we are cheered on and elevated for taking that control and putting in the work. I understand that because of this, choosing to stop dieting and not focus on your weight can feel like you are giving up on yourself.

Lifestyles are diets repackaged, which ultimately take away our health and reduce our autonomy. When I say "lifestyles," I am referring to the packages people sell you. I mean you can totally live a lifestyle in which you try to manage your health to the best of your ability, but so much of it is out of your control (more on that in Chapter 6, where we talk about social determinants of health).

But ultimately, these are "lifestyles" that don't allow you to be spontaneous and have you walking around hungry but full of fiber do backfire. It may seem like a lifestyle, but in the end, it's still a diet.

Yo-Yo Dieting

Now, I can sit here and give you stats on why diets don't work. You may not need science or research to back that up because your lived experience can tell you that. You know from experience that you go on a diet, get super restrictive, and then cannot keep it up and have to stop. You stop because life happens, because you just can't restrict carbs anymore, or because you came to the conclusion that dieting was stupid. Simple as that. But as soon as you stop, the weight you lost comes back, and then some. This is what we call the binge-restrict cycle, weight cycling, or yo-yo dieting, which is a pattern of losing weight, regaining it, and then dieting again. This cyclical loss and gain of weight can have detrimental effects on your physical and mental health.

I'm sure many of you have been through this, and quite frankly, I think it's pure insanity and not good for your health. Our bodies will automatically do anything to stay alive, so when you're dieting, your body assumes you are in a famine and slows down your metabolism to conserve energy. That means fewer calories burned or utilized for energy. Once your body is conserving energy, you regain weight quicker and your body stores it in your abdomen as visceral fat, a kind of fat that wraps around your organs. People in many body sizes can have visceral fat, and it should not be confused with having subcutaneous belly fat just below the skin. A high level of visceral fat can increase your risk of health problems such as hypertension, heart disease, and type 2 diabetes.

Yo-yo dieting leads to more stress. It can also lead to going through periods of restriction and bingeing, and increases your risk of developing eating disorders. It impacts your mental health and can lead to depression and anxiety as well as low self-esteem. The more your diets "fail," the more you think something is wrong with you. But the truth is, nothing is wrong with you, and diets are meant to fail and the only reason you keep going back is because they tell you, *Well, if it didn't work, it's your fault because we gave you the tools.* The tools are flawed and causing you harm because your body and brain are fighting what you're doing to yourself just to stay freaking alive and produce energy.

It is wrong to put the burden on you when a diet doesn't work. We're taught to expect that our bodies can (and should) function with less with no risk of future weight regain. The tools we are given are unsustainable, and this is what keeps you coming back to the same restrictive diet or a different one. You continue to restrict yourself to prevent or reduce weight gain, which keeps you on a hamster wheel of living by the diet.

It's important to highlight that if you begin performing healthy behaviors and your body changes as a result of incorporating movement and positive nutrition, this is not bad. It is neutral. So many chulas who I see say they feel extreme guilt when they lose weight unintentionally because they think that means they are back in diet culture. Your weight is not a behavior, so if you lose weight because you added healthy behaviors, why would that be diet culture? Weight is a neutral biomarker for me. Whether it goes up, goes down, or stays the same, that is not what I focus on. I focus on the behaviors and especially the nutrition because that is my job. We need to understand that guilt and shame have no place in how we view ourselves.

SOCIAL MEDIA, INFLUENCERS, AND CELEBRITIES

Social media is the fucking wild, wild west when it comes to diets. Now, I understand that many of you see me as an influencer. I do not see myself this way. First and foremost, I'm a dietitian, and helping people live healthy lives is always my first goal. I'm not here for the money or the partnerships or the clout. I'm here because I have the education, professional training, and experience to inform people about how to do what's best for their bodies.

But still everything I write is questioned; I mean *everything*. I once was asked how I could say with certainty that a person with diabetes could eat white rice. My response: *My nutrition education as a registered dietitian, which taught me how to manage disease with food.* It's not lost on me that I don't fit the dietitian mold or the influencer mold. I am loud, I have wild, curly hair, I curse, I let my kids eat sugar, I eat arroz blanco con habichuelas three or four times a week, and pizza is my love language. I speak Spanglish and being Dominican is part of my identity. Bachata and reggaeton fuel me, and my Caribbean skin needs the sun like my lungs need air. I am not what people think of when they think "dietitian" or "influencer." And when I ask you all why you follow me, you all say it's because I am real. And I like that, but the truth is that if I were blond, white, and probably thinner, my messaging would not be questioned. Because white supremacy and colonization have taught us that "professional" equals white. Don't believe me? Google it. Our community has also been taught that "American" is better. The American is blond, has blue eyes, has long hair, and is beautiful.

All this is to say that I get questioned a lot. But the influencers who fit the bill, the dietitians who fit this look, and anyone who can post pictures side by side and say *Eat like me, look like me,* do not. Social media has created a world where everyone and their mom, including me, is selling you something. But unfortunately, not all programs are created equal. Many influencers and celebrities sell dangerous diets that can cause so much harm and even lead to eating disorders.

In March 2023, a well-known influencer became the first social media star to be taken to court for deceptive practices (two months later, the state and the influencer reached a $400,000 settlement) for selling dangerous workout plans and meal plans that were causing people to have disordered eating habits. She never went to trial because the case was settled, so this person was not held accountable for all the harm she caused, and eventually she rebranded herself as a Christian and still has half a million followers. That is the privilege some are afforded, while others are not.

Whereas celebrities and influencers fearmonger over even the air we breathe at this point, I hope that this book will help you to choose the tools that work for you and your family so you can live your best life. These self-professed "experts" thrive on using black-and-white thinking, all-or-nothing thoughts, and the fact that we all want to be accepted. Honestly, who wouldn't want to know the specific black-and-white answers (if they existed) to getting thin, making money, and achieving the ideal beauty standard? With compassion, let me tell you that I understand that we believe this would make life so much easier, especially nutrition and body image.

Watching these people gives us something to aspire to, but it's also dangerous. Gwyneth Paltrow went viral for saying she basically only drinks bone broth and does IV supplements to get the rest of her nutrition. It's probably one of the only times I saw TikTok and the internet come together to call out how dangerous these statements were. The message that was put out was this: *I do not eat and I live off an IV.* What an immense amount of privilege it takes to starve oneself intentionally and spend thousands of dollars on IV therapy that is "hard to get" (her words, not mine) when you can just eat. Eat enough. Eat consistently, and get variety.

According to the Feeding America website,[5] 44 million Americans are food insecure in 2022[6] while influencers and celebrities are fearmongering about food that can keep people fed. In 2022, 13 million kids went hungry. But please, Shirtless Influencer Doctor, make social media content of you going off about cereals in the supermarket aisle. (I say this sarcastically, of course, because this type of content confuses the public and creates a hierarchy of foods without considering the implications of telling people to eat foods they cannot afford and to avoid the foods they can.)

Today, diets are no longer viewed as trendy, as they were ten to fifteen years ago when SlimFast, Atkins, and WeightWatchers were all the rage. The wellness industry and corporations have caught up on the fact that diets are no longer "in," and as a result, many of these brands have rebranded themselves as "lifestyles," but still push the same restrictive shit. For example, WeightWatchers renamed themselves WW (while still promoting weight loss). Noom focuses on "behavior change," Balance365 focuses on "wellness" (but is still heavily diet driven), and Beachbody is now BODi. Now, I am going to pause right here and say that you have bodily autonomy. You are allowed to do whatever you want with your body. You are allowed to diet. You are allowed to calorie count. You are allowed to do it all. And there are people who will sell you that and make millions! But I will not, and this is why I am not rich. However, I know beyond a shadow of a doubt that if I was to sell intentional weight loss and Latine-food meal plans, and calorie-deficit programs, *oyeeee,* I would be living fancy. Pero, I do not. Because I cannot sell a lie.

Now, I know that calorie deficits and meal planning for weight loss sell. But something that I will say a million times over is *You are not a robot.* You do not plug in and out daily. You do not need to micromanage your energy. And even if you do, that does not guarantee weight loss. In a perfect world with perfect science and equipment, we might be able to pinpoint exactly how much energy you need and exactly how much you are expending to figure out the right number of calories and create the perfect meal plan so you can be at your goal weight.

But before I even move on from this statement, we need to acknowledge the fatphobia in it. Because whether we see it or not, micromanaging to this degree implies that the perfect weight is thinness, that being in a large body is bad and that we should all be striving for thinness. And for a lot of people, that is a hard pill to swallow because it takes a lot of self-awareness to deal with our inner fatphobic thoughts. I am not saying it's easy. I am not saying it all goes away magically (spoiler alert: it does not), but acknowledging this brings us closer to collective liberation.

Do people lose weight on these programs? A hundred percent. Do people gain it back? Absolutely. A review of twenty-seven previously published reports of clinical trials conducted in 2022 concluded that while participants maintained a 5 percent weight loss from their baseline weight after intervention strategies were stopped, weight regain began within thirty-six weeks. For some participants this included complete weight regain.[7] Why does this happen? We have to continue the intervention in order to fight our metabolic biology. Financial privilege and access to support can help some people maintain this. For example, celebrities have chefs and personal trainers to help them sustain a loss. We have real lives and real stress.

But for real, for real. The main question is, is your lifestyle stressing you out? Does your lifestyle stop you from enjoying the little things like going to the park and randomly stopping for ice cream because you saw a new flavor that looks bomb? Does your lifestyle make you the person who brings Tupperware to the family cookout because you can eat only certain foods? Does your lifestyle make you say no to your abuela's arepas or mami's sancocho? If your lifestyle doesn't allow you to live, chula, that is a diet.*

The scary part about these so-called "lifestyles" is that we can find a diet for basically anything. You can go on the internet and anyone with a damn phone and with literally no education is telling you how to eat. Clara Nosek, MS, RDN, aka @yourdietitianbff, summarized this concept so well in the form of a bell curve, which I've re-created below. I do, however, think it's important to note that there are real barriers to education in this country and not everyone has the opportunity to get a degree, and there are people doing really good work with no credentials. But those people aren't selling you snake oil and lies; they understand their scope of practice and stay there.

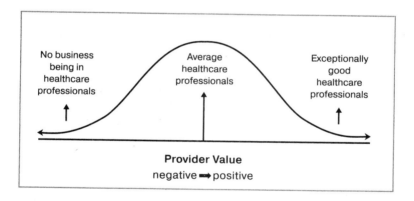

Picture this bell curve. We have exceptionally good healthcare providers, dietitians, and nutritionists who do amazing work but might not be on the internet promoting that good work. Then we

---

* Nuanced Note: And because dios sabe that nowadays we have to spell everything out because a troll will come out of the woodwork and say, *BUT I am allergic to gluten,* or *I can't have xyz.* Bestie, then this paragraph was not for you. If you are allergic to or dislike a food, *do not eat it.*

have the average ones, the majority. And then the ones who have no business practicing. Unfortunately, the ones on that end are the loudest and become viral. They are the ones who spew ridiculous diets, spread fear and misinformation, and have a million followers.

The journey from dieting, to dieting on the DL, to truly unlearning diets is founded on education. If you feel like you're Yocayra going from diet to diet for the sake of your health, learning what food terms mean ("organic," "pesticides," "clean eating," "macros") is the first step to letting go of the black-and-white thinking that's keeping you in the diet game. We have to undo the idea that eating perfectly is going to magically provide us with health and the absence of sickness. In many ways, perfectionism keeps us trapped, but understanding our food can help our health and reduce our risk. But we need to approach this not from a place of fear, but from a place of curiosity.

Therefore, I invite you to view it in another way. If you are working on your health by sleeping better, working out regularly in ways that feel good to you, eating consistently and enough, getting variety, feeling energized, hydrating, reducing stress, and getting great lab work but your weight does not come down or goes up, will you stop those healthy behaviors? Will you go back to those old dieting ways just to try to get that number back down? If your answer is yes, then it was never truly about health, it was about the number on the scale.

Yocayra's situation is not uncommon, and people who are tired of dieting are encouraged to find a "healthy lifestyle." What it came down to was not micromanaging her life to find health, but actually embracing all the parts of her that made her feel good, including her cultural foods.

TLDR: Diet culture is insidious, and you can basically find a diet that contradicts another in any Google search. The Minnesota Starvation Experiment laid the groundwork to show us how the body reacts to restriction, and today we see the symptoms exhibited by influencers daily while they're trying to sell you a lifestyle. Despite having this information and our own lived experience with restrictive eating, yo-yo dieting, and weight cycling, we are still out here dieting and calling it a lifestyle. So take a deep breath, let go of the diets disguised as lifestyles, and let's find real health.

CHULA PRACTICE:

1. Diet culture does not get to steal healthy behaviors. You get to choose how to reduce stress, add exercise, and eat. This week, how can you add nutrition or movement or stress relief that feels good to your life?
2. Think about what is restrictive in your lifestyle. Are there any habits you've been holding on to because you've been told they're supposed to be good for you? Write them down. How are these things preventing you from living a fuller, more authentic life?

FUNDAMENTALS
OF INTUITIVE EATING

Chula Story: This One's About Me!

WELL, we have gotten to the chapter that, if you follow me, you've been waiting for because you want the chisme. For those of you who do not follow me and this is all new to you, let's talk about Intuitive Eating—how I learned about it, how I felt about it in the past, and how I feel about it now. Buckle up, chulas, we are going for a ride.

Unless you have zero social media accounts, you've probably heard of Intuitive Eating.[1] Although the book *Intuitive Eating* was first published in 1995 by Evelyn Tribole and Elyse Resch, I didn't know about it until I opened my business account on Instagram. Before finding Intuitive Eating, I called myself "anti-diet," but I truly was not. I describe it as a fork in the road, where I knew dieting was bad and restriction and calorie counting didn't work, but I still celebrated weight loss and encouraged my patients to lose 5 to 10 percent of their weight, pero not by dieting, but by portion controlling. So, I was your anti-diet dietitian who portion-controlled your white rice and beans, helped you lose weight, and celebrated your culture. And I was hardcore about it too. I mean, I was convinced I was going to cure diabetes, which I would love to do, but now I know how complicated things really are. I thought I was anti-diet because I didn't prescribe diets like keto or low carb or calorie tracking, etc. As I write this book, I recognize that this approach was not true to the anti-diet movement, which in essence means not promoting weight loss and diets on the DL.

I worked all over Philly, first for another company doing home visits. As one of the only Latina dietitians in the area who spoke Spanish, I was sent all over North Philly to work with patients with diabetes. But I slowly started to realize that I could talk to these people until I was blue in the face, but they were not going to drink kale smoothies or eat brown rice (which is what my old job had wanted me to promote). So I started educating them in my way, and I realized that people will eat and care about nutrition when the food is something they know and understand. At Penn State, I had already questioned nutrition recommendations a lot, to the point where I got kicked out of a class for being loud and unruly when someone said they didn't understand why parents fed their kids McDonald's. News flash: Because sometimes that is the only thing available in our communities. Then my adviser told me that I would never make it as a dietitian because I wanted to work in the Latine community, and that I would fail because no one in the community listens. Basically, we were taught that community nutrition, which involves working directly with communities of people who are at or below the poverty line and/or with people of color, is essentially "not worth it." My adviser reminded me that these communities have a lot of "noncompliance," meaning that they don't follow through on what you teach them, making it a waste of time. According to professors like one I had named Diane, people in these communities just don't listen or care about their health. But I knew in my corazon that I wanted to work with my people so they could watch and learn from someone who looked like them. Hi, Diane! Look, I made it!

Basically, I always questioned the nutrition information I learned because it was so stereotyped. I never questioned the science—the Krebs cycle is the Krebs cycle (learning these metabolism cycles still gives me nightmares). I never questioned that carbs, proteins, and fats have enzymes and mechanisms in place that allow them to be digested by our bodies. I do, however, question dietitians who have the same science background as me and sell keto, but that is for another book. I quickly realized that my family ate arroz con habichuelas daily and no one was sick. I knew my parents' friends in DR ate platanos and malanga and were thriving. Therefore, I lived with a lot of dissonance. But, as I always say, as a first-gen Dominican American, the first in my family to go to college, I was not going to fuck shit up and question things. I was raised to stay quiet, to listen, and to respect. Respecting elders and established systems was instilled in me at a young age. When I was in school, this meant that I was not going to question my teachers or professors even if I wanted to. When I did do this, I was reprimanded, which further reinforced my need to respect the system in order to participate in it.

As I pursued my education at a white institution, I would not question my professors. I thought, *They must be right.* And so, when I say it takes a lot of critical thinking to wipe that much white supremacy from our minds, I mean it. Because you are paying a shit ton of money to learn, and if that professor says white rice and beans are what are causing the Latino community to have higher rates of diabetes, you believe it and you educate others on that. But that never sat well with me, and I took it upon myself to get answers because the math was not mathing.

I also want to raise a red flag about my education as a dietitian, not the science stuff where I learned how the body breaks down food, but the counseling part and how to speak to the BIPOC communities, and specifically, my Latine community. In an article on her Substack titled "The Unspoken History of Early Dietitians and Eugenics,"[2] my fellow dietitian Anjali Prasertong discusses Lenna Frances Cooper, one of the founders of the Academy of Nutrition and Dietetics, who was known to be a friend of the Kellogg family. Prasertong quotes a passage from the book *The Secret History of Home Economics,* by Danielle Dreilinger, in which she describes Cooper's lifestyle:

> She believed in long walks, no makeup, eight glasses of water a day, a vegetarian diet, and the power of nutrition to transform health. . . . Every month, she suggested delicious, vegetable-heavy, seasonal dishes and explained the science behind their health benefits.

Prasertong says in her piece that Cooper was in some ways ahead of her time and ate similarly to a health food influencer. Now, as Prasertong mentions, and as I have been pointing out in discussing the Minnesota Starvation Experiment, all these tendencies are eerily like those of modern-day dietitians and mommy bloggers who are selling disordered eating–filled lifestyles in the name of health. But it's not the dishes themselves or even the habits that bother me, but rather the sense of moral superiority it gives those who eat and live like this, which makes them frown upon those who do not.

Although not a eugenicist herself, Cooper worked closely with some who were. There's no record of her speaking up against eugenics or the idea that eating a certain way makes you morally superior, which her colleague John Harvey Kellogg firmly believed. It makes me wonder what Cooper, the cofounder of my profession, would think about the way I counsel my patients to embrace their cultural foods or even the way I feed my own children. To her, eating a plate of mangu might have been "savage," "unhealthy," full of fat, and wrong. Consequently, dietitians who did not grow up eating mangu would probably be biased to think the same because they aren't taught to see the nutrition and fiber in a platano, the nutrients in pickled onions, or the fat in the cheese and salami that helps us absorb it all.

As dietitians, we are taught to counsel a certain way and to discuss strategies that promote certain styles of eating. We cannot ignore the roots of the profession and the type of thinking that informed our education. Looking back on Prasertong's Substack, I get curious about how much of my education is based on food morality.

Working as a community nutritionist before I sat for my registration exam helped me see just how much of our culture is erased from dietetics and public health spaces. There are curriculums to be followed, handouts to give out, and preapproved lessons you can't deviate from. I had to educate as best I could while having to contradict MyPlate's brown-rice-over-white-rice recommendation to health centers in Black and Brown communities because I had to follow the rules. I've seen other BIPOC nutritionists speak to their BIPOC clients with an arrogance that says "I'm better than you are now" and "I can save you from your own choices." Because these nutritionists got an education, they think they have the power to tell everyone exactly what to do to be like them, never once questioning what it is they're preaching to their own communities. In so many ways, this approach is just the same as being in school and not questioning your teachers.

Therefore, do I get sad when I see BIPOC dietitians, especially Latine dietitians, spreading the whitewashed nutrition education we learned? Yes. But I know that they have to put in the work to want to learn a new and different way, and oftentimes unconscious and conscious biases plus money speak louder than doing the right thing. As of 2022, only 13 percent of dietitians identify as Latine. If we were to break that down, I'd bet that many, if not the majority, were likely able to pass as white, which means that there is comfort and acceptance in upholding these ideals. Again, I'm not knocking them, but that is not the truth I stand in. I want to dismantle the bullshit and teach real nutrition. So, when I went out looking for answers, I found Intuitive Eating. I immediately bought the book and read it.

It was the first time in my career that I had words to describe what I knew was right—that eating doesn't have to be complicated, and neither does nutrition. Once I started my IG account, Intuitive Eating dietitians started popping up all over my feed.

In 2018, about five years into my being a dietitian, Alissa Rumsey, MS, RD, CSCS, hosted an event for dietitians in NYC. I applied for a scholarship and won. I went to NYC ready to learn, but even then, I was still at that fork in the road where I wholeheartedly believed that losing weight intentionally was worth supporting and that I could help others achieve that. But as a result of this event, I started to reconsider my approach. The seed that was planted at Alissa's event then grew roots at my first Weight Inclusive Nutrition and Dietetics conference in Washington, D.C., that same year, hosted by Heather Caplan, RDN. Heather is the founder of Weight Inclusive Nutrition and Dietetics [WIND], which is a community and platform for educating nutrition professionals from an anti-diet lens.

I remember taking the train alone to D.C. and not knowing anyone at the conference. I stayed for the weekend to attend the full event. I remember how stressed I was because I had left my baby boy for the first time overnight. I remember not knowing what to expect. I had no clue what I was getting myself into, but I took the chance. When I got there, the room was set up with round tables, and I took a seat in the far-right corner, toward the back. I sat through all the research presentations by Dr. Kendrin Sonneville, ScD, RDN. She discussed weight stigma and weight-loss research. Dr. Sonneville started her presentation and had us put our hands under the table and we began the "put a finger down" activity. Members of the audience were asked to put a finger down if we had ever had trouble fitting into an airplane seat, if we had ever had issues sitting in a roller-coaster seat, and the list went on. I never put a finger down because my size is acceptable to society, and that was the first time in my life that I really understood fatphobia.

For a full weekend, I had to sit in the suckiness of knowing how much harm (unintentionally of course) I was causing my patients. This is when I started to unlearn a lot of what dietetics had taught me to be "right" (such as portion control) and really began to take a patient-centered approach. I left D.C. after that weekend and never looked back. I immersed myself in reading all the books I recommended in Chapter 1 and attended as many conferences as I could. That weekend changed the dietitian I was forever.

I decided to work on my Intuitive Eating certification. These principles had given me the words to explain what I had always thought about nutrition but wasn't taught in my education. In my business, it became my new branding—what I was all about. But as I learned and evolved, I started seeing the connections among nutrition, fat liberation, racial justice, anti-fatness, and anti-blackness. It all exploded even more during the summer of 2020, when the leaders of these movements were in the forefront teaching and many of us were truly listening, not just putting black squares° up on Instagram.

° You probably recall people at that time posting black squares in solidarity with Black Lives Matter. For many, this was an easy way to participate in a movement without there being much accountability for changed behavior and thinking.

Soon after that, I began to see a shift. Many of the accounts that I had looked up to were not focusing on these real issues like anti-fat bias, racism, and food insecurity, and they continued to move along like these systemic issues didn't affect the people they were working with, and continued to move along like these systemic issues had nothing to do with Intuitive Eating. Many of them said that politics did not need to be and should not be involved. Prominent Intuitive Eating accounts with large followings doubled down on saying that food isn't political and continued to post reminders to "Just eat the donut" instead of pushing forward nutrition knowledge and cultural context. I argued that there was more to gain in posting cheeky videos about binge eating and "eating the cookie without fear" than there was for dietitians to use their privilege and educate about systemic issues on our nutrition. I started to feel like Intuitive Eating was being marketed to white women with privilege because that's both easier and doesn't require you to name the underlying influences on our nutrition.

I realized that IE is not for white women only, and it's not a permission slip to eat the donut. It is more than that, but the more I saw the owners of these accounts act as though people who look like me didn't deserve to be treated with dignity and respect, the more I wanted to distance myself from the movement. In addition, many nutrition accounts started selling Intuitive Eating techniques alongside the promise of weight loss, which was a sign that the movement was becoming further co-opted and even more distanced from its original purpose.

The more that this happened, the more I emphasized nutrition about how our foods, culture, and tradition are all nourishing. It truly fueled me to continue to do this work without having to always label myself as an "Intuitive Eating dietitian." I knew that being a Latina dietitian who could embrace the gray and the nuance was the hole I needed to fill.

I think that's why when I started posting, my community felt so seen. I hadn't seen another Latina dietitian active on social media posting about Intuitive Eating, and many learned about it from me, which was amazing. And from the very beginning I talked about the lack of culture, and that certainly resonated.

After realizing that IE was not going to be enough for my community, I decided not to finish my coursework to become a certified Intuitive Eating dietitian. It did not feel right to do so; it felt like I couldn't be myself and call out the issues. I worried that it would pigeonhole me. In addition, in the IE world, I am still othered. There are huge IE accounts that are super problematic but are never called out. Yet I post about the difference between white rice and brown rice and I get destroyed in the comments. There have been so many occasions when one of my BIPOC dietitian friends or I post something innocent like *Eat white rice* and we get the worst comments, but then one of these bigger accounts mimics our post and the comments are all *Omg you're so great* and *I never thought of this before.* But what hurts the most is that the hate comes from our own dietetics community, and you can see clearly how unconscious bias can be so pervasive. For many people, white equals right while black or brown equals wrong.

Intuitive Eating was written by two very smart white women, but it's still missing sazón and nuance. Although the framework of IE is used for those with eating disorders and in disordered-eating recovery, I don't want us to miss those who are, and were, food insecure, and the BIPOC community that has had so much stolen from it, because they deserve health too. Our Latine community deserves to find health on our terms, and we don't always need labels. We need to learn, and we need to heal.

My biggest fears and concerns revolve around the potential distortion of Intuitive Eating. With the rise in its popularity, the message can sometimes get lost or misconstrued. It's important to approach this practice with authenticity, to seek out the right educators and sources, and to remember that Intuitive Eating, like many wellness practices, is not a one-size-fits-all solution. While some may adopt all its principles, others might find that they only need to work on some principles. The overall goal is to discover what genuinely serves and nourishes your unique self.

Here, I've broken down the ten principles of the Intuitive Eating framework so we can first understand the basics of this approach.

IE Principle	Intended Meaning	A Sprinkle of Sazón
Reject the Diet Mentality	Dismantle beliefs around dieting and acknowledge that diets have failed you. Unfollow accounts that make you feel bad. Diversify your social media feed.	It's important to dismantle diet culture, but it's also important to understand the racism and white supremacy attached to it and how these negative forces affect the BIPOC community specifically. If we don't understand how BMI and nutrition have always been white-washed, we cannot understand how health standards now were not made for us. When we see it through this lens, it allows us to fully reject diets.
Honor Your Hunger	Reclaim power by nourishing yourself and listening to your needs. Use the hunger scale, a tool for nuancing your hunger and fullness cues, to gauge your hunger levels.	The hunger scale is awesome, but it's often used as a diet. Using nuance and discussing how culture and food affect our hunger is important. Culturally, we are taught to be afraid of our hunger, and we need to reclaim it.

IE Principle	Intended Meaning	A Sprinkle of Sazón
Make Peace with Food	Allow yourself to eat without guilt. Jump off the binge-restrict cycle and focus on your needs.	It's so important to learn to eat with intention and connection. So is understanding the binge-restrict cycle and unlearning the unspoken rules in many of our cultures that tell us we are "letting ourselves go" when we eat. Coping with the pressure to fit the Latina ideal is hard, but unlearning it is possible.
Challenge the Food Police	Challenge ingrained food rules and see nutrition differently. Unlearn myths like "Don't eat carbs" and "Don't eat after 6 P.M."	Our mamis and abuelas have taught us a lot of food rules, and so has society. Unlearning them takes some critical thinking and self-discovery. Many of the diets we do increase our risk for the chronic conditions we often are trying to run away from.
Discover Satisfaction	Eat food that is not just nourishing but also satisfying and enjoyable. Realize that it's not just about calories in and calories out.	Food is meant to taste delicioso. Your meals are supposed to be like a big hug from your abuela. It's meant to bring you close to your culture and traditions. We want to reduce stress and find pleasure in it again. This is an important part of this journey.
Feel Your Fullness	Understand and appreciate the sensation of fullness. Learn to recognize when you are full or not full enough.	Understanding fullness and setting boundaries with our familia is key, but a simple "no" sometimes does not work in our communities and we need to recognize and figure out how to deal with that when it happens.

IE Principle	Intended Meaning	A Sprinkle of Sazón
Cope with Emotions with Kindness	Understand that using food as a coping mechanism is normal, but also find other ways to cope.	Understanding that food is a perfectly fine coping mechanism is key; we never want to become numb to it. And we need to create other ways to cope with food that are significant for us.
Respect Your Body	Learn to respect yourself regardless of your size.	Latine culture often teaches us that our bodies are not ours, and we become so disconnected from them. We need to learn to respect our bodies, to learn about the diversity in bodies, to undo a lot of the colonization and novela culture behind how we view our cuerpos.
Joyful Movement	Maintain a balanced relationship with exercise that works for you.	Unlearning rules around exercise is hard. But learning how it can help us reduce our risk for chronic disease is important. Finding movement that works for you is key. Dance that bachata, chula.
Gentle Nutrition	Focus on adding nutrients to your diet and managing chronic conditions without being overly restrictive.	Honor your culture, health, and nutrition: It is key that we learn how our cultural foods fit the nutrition guidelines and nourish us. We do not have to change our recipes to fight chronic disease, and we can easily add more cultural ingredients to our day that can help us find authentic health.

THE PROS AND CONS OF INTUITIVE EATING

Like I said, IE helped me find the words and tools I needed to fully embrace the dietitian I feel I was meant to be, and I am forever thankful for that. But let's review how Intuitive Eating is not the only right way to eat. It has both pros and cons.

PROS

For me, there are four major pros to Intuitive Eating. When utilized correctly, these principles can be powerful tools for taking back your life—you'll be able to see the end of the tunnel when it comes to dieting. The pros of Intuitive Eating are:

1. **You learn to break away from the diet mentality and guilt over food.** This is why so many people are drawn to the Intuitive Eating lens. We all know diets do not work, so trying to find an alternative that helps you break away from that feels so freaking freeing. We want to eat in peace without stressing about every crumb.

2. **It allows for pleasure and enjoyment of food without shame and guilt.** Finding joy in eating is so important, and it's another reason so many people are drawn to this framework. This is why you see those IG posts of dietitians eating cookies, ha ha. Because you should be able to. And you should also be able to eat *all* your cultural foods without guilt. You should feel all the feels of biting into a warm arepa. It should feel good and enjoyable.

3. **You'll reconnect with your body and its cues.** You should be able to understand your body and its needs. IE helps with that connection with hunger and fullness so you no longer fear them but rather learn to truly nourish your body.

4. **You'll learn to emphasize flexibility and individual needs.**

This is why I really love this lens. It's all about finding what works for you and only you. Learning your preferences and having flexibility to eat in a way that honors your health is *key*. You should have the flexibility to figure this all out and be able to evolve and know what your body needs no matter what crap the world throws at you.

Additionally, I think it's important to take a moment and talk about the Health at Every Size (HAES) Principles and Framework of Care and how they function hand in hand with Intuitive Eating. While I was in the middle of learning IE, I, like many other RDs, was also introduced to the HAES approach to providing healthcare to fat people that doesn't focus on losing weight. Incorporating those principles into my own work was a way to bring in that social justice piece that had become important to me. When I realized that the principles of Intuitive Eating don't incorporate social justice, it was obvious to me that this is essential if we want to create substantial change in our communities.

HAES[3] IS A trademarked lens of practice created by ASDAH, the Association for Size Diversity and Health. This overseeing organization supports, promotes, and educates healthcare professionals on the HAES philosophy, which focuses on five pillars of health and giving everyone access to them no matter their size, ability, sexuality, or gender:

1. **Weight inclusivity:** HAES recognizes that bodies come in all shapes and sizes. Body diversity is real, and weight is not a reliable indicator of health or of someone's worth. HAES promotes respect for all cuerpos and so do I.
2. **Health enhancement:** HAES focuses on supporting every-

one in finding healthy behaviors that promote physical, emotional, and mental well-being instead of focusing on weight loss. It's about self-care, moving your body in joyous ways, and nourishing your body.

3. **Respectful care:** This part speaks to the medical professionals reading this. It is important to respect your patients. This means we have to provide compassionate, nonjudgmental care to all regardless of size and reject weight stigma and any practices that harm a person's health or well-being. I see you doctors who give out handouts with the words "NO WHITE FOODS" and the first thing on the list is white rice. ☹

4. **Eating for well-being:** Okay, this is my area of expertise, and seriously such an important one. I cannot tell you how many people just do not eat enough. HAES promotes a positive and balanced approach to nutrition, which means listening to your body, hunger, and fullness; not restricting; and never feeling guilty. If you have no clue what this looks like, don't you worry, because that is what this book is all about, chula.

5. **Life-enhancing movement:** Lastly, everyone needs to find movement that helps them feel good and that is within their abilities. This means gyms, parks, and recreational spaces need to provide equipment that allows people of different abilities and sizes to use it. This means as a whole society we need to be inclusive, because healthism tells us we need to move our bodies a certain way to be good or to be counted as healthy. However, when we don't because the appropriate equipment and structures aren't safe or available, the blame is placed on the individual and not the social structures.

Just like Intuitive Eating, HAES provides a framework we can utilize to be more inclusive and fat positive for our patients. Between 2022 and 2024, ASDAH updated their framework to include the following principles:

1. Grounding in liberatory frameworks
2. Patient bodily autonomy
3. Informed consent
4. Compassionate care
5. Critical analysis, application, and execution of research and medical recommendations related to weight
6. Skills and equipment to provide compassionate and comprehensive care for fat people's bodies
7. Provider roles and responsibilities
8. Tools that support well-being and healing without contributing to oppression
9. Addressing your anti-fat bias
10. Addressing systemic anti-fat bias

It is important to note that not all IE providers are HAES adherents and vice versa, but I do use both lenses in my work as needed. Just like IE, HAES cannot be the be-all and end-all. People can get religious and overzealous about it, but I want to emphasize that these should be used as *guides*, not gospel.

A few years ago, I read Amanda Montell's *Cultish: The Language of Fanaticism* along with my dietitian pal Clara Nosek. We texted back and forth about the book and then we met up in Chicago in January 2023. We were discussing how impactful we both found the book, and Clara hit me with this important distinction:

> Intuitive Eating is a great tool, but it's not *the* tool. Much like the critiques of white feminism, Intuitive Eating doesn't seek to dismantle the systems of oppression that create and uphold diet culture.

Since most dietitians who practice IE are thin, able-bodied cis women, they don't tend to discuss the systems of oppression that need to be dismantled for people to have access to food, healthcare, housing, and health. It feels as though the sole goal is to dismantle diet culture; however, we cannot dismantle diet culture if we aren't talking about dismantling white supremacy, because they are one and the same. This is why I always say that we cannot talk about health without noting that not everyone has access to the same level of health-promoting behaviors.

Clara looked at me, sighed, and added, "Unfortunately, what we see in today's application of IE is the desire to replace diet culture with a 'better' set of rules." And this point leads me to the cons about IE:

CONS

1. **It inspires fanaticism.** As Clara noted, IE often feels like a transference of one behavior to another. For some, it can become an obsession with being right—following the right way to eat and the right way to live. But in reality, no one holds the trademark on eating "right." I believe the original goal of Intuitive Eating was for it to function as a tool, to truly allow people to move past the rules-based diets created to help everyone just live (and I think Evelyn agrees with this because she has shared several of my posts about nuance and IE). But when people apply an all-or-nothing approach to IE as the best way to heal your relationship with food, it creates an almost cultlike following of believers. Dietitians, nutritionists, and followers alike can become fanatics to the point of not being able to consider any other way of eating or thinking about food. It becomes about being "right" in the world of nutrition instead of what I believe it should be all along: the practice of just being a human and eating.

2. **It's considered morally superior and better.** In a world where we must make so many decisions, it's understandable to want answers to cut through the chaos and to check off items on a list. However, this has the potential to take a holier-than-thou perspective, and this is what I see the most on social media. A message I see a lot is that if you aren't doing IE, you are wrong. If you aren't following the steps to a T, you are wrong. God forbid you should say anything about thoughts of losing weight. Excommunicated! There is zero nuance in allowing people to figure out what works for them. And unfortunately, there is a lot of gaslighting of people in bigger bodies. You can look at the hashtag and it's all thin white women holding a scale and screaming, *Just throw it away* (and I am guilty of having made this post, but again, I have learned and grown since). There's constant dismissal of the real and awful things people in fat bodies experience daily. For many people, it's not as fucking simple as throwing away the scale or eating the cookies.

3. **There's no mention of nutrition or social determinants of health.** Although gentle nutrition is technically the tenth principle, when you look at these social media accounts there isn't much talk about nutrition and never any talk about people in low-income communities being shamed for just eating the donut while these account holders are praised for eating them. There is no mention of the reasons why we don't have access to food or how health disparities affect communities of color and how many people cannot just eat when they are hungry. Many focus only on the "just eat the cookies" bit, and since there's not much sustenance to the post, people will read the caption and think, *Oh okay, I'm just going to go at it.* What ends up happening is that these people will transfer one behavior for another. A lot of chulas in my group tell me that

when they enter the "fuck it" stage without guidance, they end up bingeing and many walk away with blood sugar control issues because they didn't work with someone to help them understand how not to swing to the other end of the pendulum.

As a dietitian who does focus on nutrition, I have heard horror stories from clients who find me after working with big, notable Intuitive Eating Instagram dietitians. For example, I had someone in my six-week group who worked with an IE RD who emphasized meeting her body where it was. Sometimes for my client this meant eating whole sleeves of Oreos. When she asked the RD about nutrition, she received replies like "Your body knows what it needs" and "Give your body what it wants." She was reminded to not stress about nutrition and to eat whatever she wanted. While I agree that nutrition needs to be stress-free, what is lost here is intention and education. My client was learning to eat more food, which was great, but she was not learning how to routinely eat balanced meals that honor both her hunger and her preferences.

4. **It misses cultural nuance and perspective.** This is where I focus a lot of my time. If you are learning nutrition but it's not elevating your cultural foods, that is an issue. If your way of being an intuitive eater is by "healthifying" your foods and still bad-mouthing them, then you did not heal your relationship with food.

Someone may have been educated to switch to brown rice instead of eating white rice. This is an example of healthifying a dish—taking a dish as it is and making "healthier" swaps to decrease calories (not necessarily to add nutrition). This happens all the time in diet programs and even in advice from dietitians. Even if brown rice is not culturally appropriate for the dish, it is not uncommon to see healthifying transform into embracing the idea that "It tastes better" or "It's just as good" or "I prefer this now."

Then, when someone steps into IE, it is common for them to ask themselves, *Why do I eat certain foods?* When Intuitive Eating lacks nuance, clients can say to themselves, "No, I really do prefer brown rice" without unpacking the context surrounding this feeling. Often, we feel better making these choices because they are more acceptable socially and align with others' definition of health. Intuitive eating does not always make space for the nuance required to dig into the social influence of why we eat what we eat.

In summary, are we still using Intuitive Eating to diet or to practice whitewashed nutrition standards? Are we able to explore satisfaction with just the ten principles of IE?

The problem with IE is bigger than the framework itself. It has to do with the way our world operates. According to a poll of two thousand individuals, the average person will adopt 126 diets in their lifetime.[4] That is so many different rules, decisions, programs, and protocols. When it comes time to think about intuitively eating, people are overwhelmed. So much of life is uncontrollable, yet food can almost always be controlled with a diet. Intuitive eating can feel like going from one extreme to another. As a result, I see clients and followers approach IE as gospel instead of as a flexible mindset. It becomes a new set of rules and a community with right and wrong decision-making. It can feel like a cult.

In her book *Cultish*, Amanda Montell[5] explains why modern cultish groups can be so compelling:

> They help alleviate the anxious mayhem of living in a world that presents almost too many possibilities for who to be (or at least the illusion of such). . . . For most of America's history,

there were comparatively few directions a person's career, hobbies, place of residence, romantic relationships, diet, aesthetic—everything—could easily go in. But the twenty-first century presents folks (those of some privilege, that is) with a Cheesecake Factory–size menu of decisions to make. The sheer quantity can be paralyzing, especially in an era of radical self-creation. . . . As our generational lore goes, millennials' parents told them they could grow up to be whatever they wanted, but then that cereal aisle of endless "what ifs" and "could bes" turned out to be so crushing, all they wanted was a guru to tell them which to pick.

When you think about eating using Intuitive Eating, it can feel like it has calmness and structure but allotted flexibility to eat in a world that has so many damn food rules, and I agree with that. Intuitive Eating can certainly provide us with this calmness, but unfortunately people often take it to the fanaticism end. A simple example here is the idea that you can't have diet soda because that would mean you're on a diet. I've also witnessed others (and myself) getting criticized for posting nutrition content. Clients approach my nutrition resource library with skepticism—*Isn't this dieting? Adding fiber is dieting, isn't it?* Talking about nutrition feels like dieting to them, which is at the fanatical end of IE. There is also hyperfixation on Intuitive Eating being the only right way. I have seen content that fixates on IE as the answer, even for folks who do want to lose weight. This ignores a person's autonomy and the fact that living in a smaller body might be safer (from a discrimination perspective) for some folks.

IE is put forward as the solution to all of your problems: If you do it right, you will be happy. If you aren't happy, you did it wrong. Unfortunately, this makes no space for folks to be unhappy *and* navigate their body after recovery or weight gain.

Another social media behavior I see a lot is removing comments that argue against the post or promote IE. As a creator of color, I experience inappropriate comments constantly and I do delete harmful and damaging ones, but that's not the same as deleting a comment because the person doesn't agree with your sales point—that comes from a place of needing to be "right" on all things.

It's normal to learn new things and change your mind based on findings you didn't have before. Evolving requires adaptation! We are changed by the new information we receive. You could be fully immersed in dieting and feel like it's The Only Way, but with new information, you can make better decisions for your health and wellness. On the other hand, you may see IE as The Only Way to freedom and peace with food, but it's much more nuanced than that. And if reading this bothers you, I think you really need to reevaluate your relationship with Intuitive Eating.

TLDR: IE is just a tool. It doesn't make you morally superior. It isn't the gospel or the *only* way to eat. IE is not an end goal you can achieve by checking off a list of ten principles. IE has the potential to help you heal from previous dieting experiences so you feel better.

CHULA PRACTICE:

1. If you haven't already, familiarize yourself with the ten principles of Intuitive Eating. Identify one principle you want to bring into your life for the purpose of supporting your relationship with food.
2. Consider how you can add some sazón to the principle you chose.
3. Audit the social media nutrition accounts you're following to see if you could benefit from getting more nuance, maybe even from Intuitive Eating accounts! Some of my favorites are below:

Shana Minei Spence, MS, RDN, CDN

Jasmine Westbrooks, MS, RD, LDN, CDCES, and
  Ashley Carter, RD, LDN, at EatWell Exchange

Clara Nosek, MS, RDN

Jessica Wilson, MS, RD

Dr. Whitney Trotter, DNP, APRN, PNP-BC, RDN

Zariel Grullon, RDN, CDN

Maria Sylvester Terry, MS, RDN, LDN

4

RESPECTING LA CULTURA

Chula Story: Eva

EVA is thirty-three and an engineer. She lives in Orlando with her dog and husband, and both Eva and her husband love to cook Puerto Rican dishes. At her most recent doctor's appointment, Eva was told she was prediabetic based on one slightly elevated reading, so the doctor gave her guidelines with nutritional information that said "no white carbs or starchy veggies," meaning that all root vegetables were out the window and off the table. For Eva, this meant she couldn't cook the cultural Puerto Rican staples that are actually loaded with nutrition, like yuca and yautia. When Eva first joined my private community called the Chula Club, she had had no nutrition education and was feeling like she'd have to restrict her food intake. But what she learned would help change her perspective.

In September 2022, I received an email inviting me to attend the White House Conference on Hunger, Nutrition, and Health. I was pretty shocked because I had no clue how or why I was put on this list, but I went. The conference was aimed at figuring out how the United States can combat issues around hunger, nutrition, and health. As a dietitian, I wanted to be there to hear the plan, and it would turn out to be the first time I ever heard so much talk about social determinants of health and how the BIPOC community is impacted by poverty, weight stigma, and inadequate access to healthcare. I was nervous about attending, but I was even more excited about the enlightened conversations I would be having with healthcare professionals from across the country.

Throughout the conference, I kept feeling glimmers of hope that progress could be made, but I didn't want to get my hopes up too much. The last item on the agenda that day was meeting in breakout tables. At my table was the deputy director of the U.S. Department of Agriculture. We got to talking about my work as a registered dietitian and they invited me to connect via Zoom a few weeks later to discuss my perspective on MyPlate.

MyPlate is a nutrition tool designed to help people create balanced meals. I was excited to share my culturally sensitive viewpoint on how to make this more applicable to communities of color because we do not eat brown rice, steamed chicken, and broccoli every night. I logged into the meeting on an October afternoon to join three women who worked for the USDA. I was introduced by a woman who exclaimed that meeting me was the highlight of the White House conference for her. I felt welcomed and excited, but I knew I could not give them all my ideas without knowing whether I'd be compensated for my consultation services. I shared my perspective on why MyPlate wasn't yet a household name for Latine families. I could feel the energy of the meeting change as I spoke. The women in the meeting responded defensively. It quickly turned into an uncomfortable situation because I don't believe they expected me to name the problems without providing concrete solutions. It was clear that they only wanted to pick my brain and were not happy with my contrary views on nutrition and MyPlate.

After the call, I followed up not once but four different times. The USDA ghosted me! It felt as though they wanted my knowledge for free, but I was not willing to provide that. Instead, I created a TikTok playlist for my followers about how we could change MyPlate to be more culturally appropriate for BIPOC communities. It was important to me that I share my perspective with the public in my own words and in the way I intended.

I've always held a deep appreciation for MyPlate because of its clear visual representation and organization. At its core, MyPlate serves as a tangible guide, enabling individuals to set up their plates in a manner that provides a complete and balanced meal. The tool's design allows one to see the different food groups and learn about their nutritional significance. In a world where nutritional literacy is surprisingly low, such tools can be invaluable. I've encountered numerous adults throughout my professional journey who lack basic knowledge about fundamental nutritional concepts like what carbs, proteins, and fats are. While some do have a vague understanding, the complexities of many foods remain puzzling to them.

MyPlate was introduced in 2011. It was designed as a revamped nutritional guideline—replacing the old Food Guide Pyramid—with the active involvement and endorsement of the then–first lady, Michelle Obama. Those who grew up in the 1990s might fondly remember the Food Guide Pyramid adorning the walls of health classrooms. I was happy that the pyramid was gone, as it never quite made sense to me. MyPlate was introduced as a more intuitive model aiming to provide a straightforward visual guide to balanced eating, and I enjoy using it as an educational tool.

The teachings of MyPlate aren't directed at any single institution or demographic. Various entities, from schools to nonprofits, have integrated its guidelines into their curricula. When I worked with nonprofit organizations funded by USDA grants, MyPlate was a pivotal educational tool used to teach the community nutritional guidelines. Its simplicity and effectiveness in conveying information made it easy to use in settings from the kindergarten classroom all the way through to the community kitchen.

However, as with any model, MyPlate has flaws. One of my primary concerns is the tool's limited representation of cultural foods. Many traditional dishes don't fit neatly into the segmented plate model MyPlate lays out. Without proper context and education, communities might mistakenly view their traditional foods as unhealthy or otherwise not adhering to recommended guidelines. The segmented design can suggest fixed portion sizes, potentially instilling a sense of guilt in those who desire seconds or have the need for bigger portions. Such a rigid interpretation can be detrimental to one's relationship with food. And that is where I see the most issues.

It's essential to emphasize the inherent flexibility of tools like MyPlate. Humans are diverse, with fluctuating needs and appetites. As I frequently point out, we aren't robots that plug in and out daily. On some days you might be hungrier, while on other days you might naturally just want less. The key takeaway is that MyPlate, like Intuitive Eating, is adaptable. It's a guideline, not an unyielding rule, and it should be adjusted to resonate with individual needs and circumstances.

As you can see, MyPlate[1] separates your plate into sections for the five food groups. Let's break them down together.

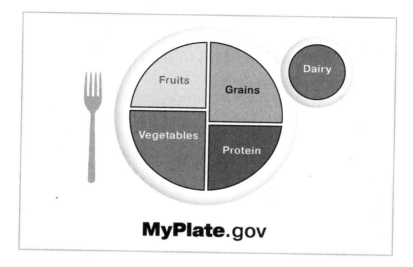

MyPlate.gov

MAKE A QUARTER OF YOUR PLATE GRAINS

In the top-right corner you will find the grains section. Grains and carbs are essentially the same, and I think this can be so confusing for those who don't have a proper education on nutrition. Many people just don't know what carbs truly are, and there is so much misinformation out there. People fear carbs, as though the macronutrient will somehow give them diabetes. News flash: It won't. Diabetes is a complex chronic condition and eating carbs will not cause it.

In the United States, there is a *huge* emphasis on wheat. We grow it here—I get it. But there are twenty-two whole grains listed on the Oldways Whole Grains Council website, including corn (yes, corn is a whole grain), amaranth, barley, oats, quinoa, and so many more. Whole wheat isn't the only one, yet when we look at the recommendations, it's basically the only one we see.

Okay, so we are making a quarter of our plate grains (reminder:

only half of your daily grains need to be whole), but in my humble opinion, when we only say "grains," we leave out carbohydrates that come from starchy veggies and fruits like potatoes and platanos. And yes, fruits and vegetables have their own section on the plate, but root veggies have an important role to play in our cultural nutrition. For the average Latine client this is confusing, because leaving out starchy veggies and fruits leaves out many cultural dishes that potentially have a lot of fiber and nutrients. If I was in charge, I would name this section "carbs" and take the fear of carbs right out of it, despite what the keto people will tell you. And why do we as dietitians and healthcare providers want you to eat whole grains? Because of the fiber, vitamins, and minerals in those whole grains. But you know what else also has these? Root veggies!

Carbohydrates are one of the three main macronutrients found in food, alongside proteins and fats. They are a crucial source of energy for our bodies. Carbohydrates come in various forms, including sugars, starches, and fibers. They are found in a wide range of foods such as grains (e.g., rice, bread), fruits, vegetables, legumes (e.g., beans, lentils), and dairy products.

When we eat carbohydrates, our bodies break them down into a type of sugar called glucose. Glucose is fuel for our cells—it provides energy the body needs to function properly. Think of glucose as the energy that powers our daily activities, from living, breathing, walking, and talking to more intense physical activities.

Once carbohydrates are digested and glucose is released into the bloodstream, the body uses it in a few different ways:

1. **For immediate energy:** Some glucose is immediately used by our cells for energy. It provides the quick fuel needed for our muscles to move, our brain to think, and our organs to work.
2. **For stored energy:** Excess glucose that our body doesn't

need for immediate energy gets stored in the liver and muscles as glycogen. Glycogen acts as a reserve for later use.

3. **For sustained energy:** When our body needs energy between meals or during prolonged activities, it can convert stored glycogen back into glucose. This process helps maintain a steady supply of energy for our body.

It's important to remember that carbohydrates themselves are not inherently bad or unhealthy. In fact, they are an essential part of a balanced diet. Carbohydrates provide important nutrients, vitamins, minerals, and fiber that the body needs to function optimally, which is why I can never, ever, ever understand how someone who has a science degree or has ever studied nutrition can push the keto diet. Yet again, the goal of many "influencers"— doctors, dietitians, healthcare providers—is to shrink you, not help you with your actual health. If it was about health, they would never push keto or many of the super-restrictive diets.

So instead of fearing carbohydrates, it's more helpful to understand their role as a vital source of energy for the body. When Eva learned this, her whole life changed. She was able to reintroduce those root veggies she had been so afraid of because she now understood the nutrients they provide. Making choices and adding nutrition to her daily meals with dishes she knew and grew up with not only reduced her stress level, it also helped her reduce her blood sugar. Let's learn about the starchy root veggies in Eva's traditional dishes and ours.

- **Yuca (cassava):** Yuca is often used in dishes like yuca fries, boiled yuca, or yuca-based doughs for empanadas or tamales. Friendly reminder: Raw yuca is poisonous, although if you ever tried to eat raw yuca, you might have broken a tooth or two trying. I think our ancestors learned this . . . quickly!

- **Batata (sweet potato):** Did you know that a batata *is* a sweet potato? We all know that the wellness world *loves* sweet potatoes, which are widely used in Latin American cuisine. But why don't we talk about all the amazing dishes that use them and how nourishing they are? It's because once again no one is translating ingredients and looking at them from a nutritional standpoint, they are just sticking to stereotypes of and biases about our foods. They can be roasted, mashed, or used in stews, soups, and various side dishes.
- **Ñame (yam):** Ñames are often used in soups or stews or roasted as a side dish.
- **Malanga:** Malanga is commonly used in Latin America and the Caribbean. Think of how you would prepare a potato. You can boil these or fry them, mash them, serve them under a stew, prepare them as chips, or enjoy them on their own.
- **Taro root:** Known as yautia blanca in the Dominican Republic, taro root is used in Latin American cooking. It is often included in soups, stews, and traditional dishes like sancocho or sopa de ocumo.
- **Papa (potato):** While potatoes are not technically root vegetables, they are widely used in Latin American cooking. They can be included in various dishes and prepared in many ways, such as boiling or frying.

Platanos, or plantains, are technically fruits. They are often grouped with the starchy root vegetables due to their culinary uses and similarities to other starchy roots. Plantains are an integral part of Latin American cuisine, and a versatile ingredient for use in both savory and sweet dishes.

- **Green plantains:** When plantains are green and unripe, they are starchy and less sweet. They are commonly used in savory dishes like tostones or patacones, when they are sliced, fried, and then mashed or flattened. I took my mom to a Peruvian restaurant and explained that patacones are tostones and she learned something that day. I can't get over how amazing it is that we all use the same ingredients in such diverse ways.

- **Yellow plantains:** As plantains ripen and turn yellow, they become softer and sweeter. Yellow plantains are often used in dishes such as maduros, for which they are fried until caramelized and served as a sweet and savory side.

All of these amazing starchy veggies should be considered carbs because they provide us with those carbohydrates rather than providing mostly fiber, vitamins, and minerals like other vegetables. Including them in this section can reduce the stigma and guilt that people feel about eating carbs. Additionally, because of their nutrient complexity, they are a great way to help reduce blood sugar.

Let's talk about the nutrition of both whole grains and root veggies, and I'll show you that smaller portions of many root veggies actually have more of these nutrients than whole grains do.

- **Carbohydrates:** Both whole grains and root vegetables provide carbohydrates, which are an important source of energy.
- **Fiber:** While whole grains may be touted as the only way to get fiber from carbs, root vegetables can also contribute to your daily fiber intake. For example, sweet potatoes, beets, and carrots contain dietary fiber that promotes digestive health, aids in satiety, and supports overall gut health. Including a variety of root vegetables in your diet can help diversify your fiber sources.
- **Vitamins and minerals:** Both whole grains and root vegetables offer a range of essential vitamins and minerals. Whole

grains such as quinoa and rice are excellent sources of B vitamins, magnesium, and zinc. On the other hand, root vegetables provide nutrients like beta-carotene (which your body converts into vitamin A), vitamin C, potassium, and other antioxidants (see below). Incorporating root vegetables and platanos into your diet alongside whole grains can ensure you're getting a variety of vitamins and minerals.

- **Antioxidants:** Root vegetables such as beets and carrots are rich in antioxidants like beta-carotene and other phytonutrients, which are nutrients obtained from plants. These compounds help protect your cells from damage caused by free radicals (unstable atoms that naturally form in your body), potentially reducing the risk of chronic diseases. Including antioxidant-rich root vegetables in your meals alongside whole grains can provide a wider range of protective nutrients.

- **Versatility and flavor:** Root vegetables, as well as platanos, offer versatility and diverse flavors. They can be roasted, boiled, fried, or incorporated into a variety of dishes, adding depth and character to your meals.

And let's not forget the cultural significance that root vegetables such as yuca hold in many countries, like the Dominican Republic, where mi familia is from. In addition, though it is technically a fruit, the plantain is used culinarily as a starchy root vegetable and prepared in many different ways. Our foods deserve to be on our plates and not villainized, which is why I take so much pride in educating people about the nutritious value of these foods.

Now, I'm going to break down the actual nutrition in a few key root veggies pa que sepan and also so you feel good about them. Remember both that the amount of nutrients you get depends on the amount you eat and that you aren't eating them alone but rather with other foods as part of a meal.

- **Yuca:** Cassava contains fiber, vitamin C, thiamine (B_1), potassium, magnesium, niacin (B_3), vitamin B_6, folate (B_9), riboflavin (B_2), zinc, and phosphorus.
- **Malanga/yautia:** This root vegetable provides fiber and some protein, along with B vitamins, vitamins A and C, magnesium, phosphorus, iron, and calcium. I have actually started seeing yautia chips in hipster areas (again, when the dominant white culture decides it's healthy, we start seeing it in trendy restaurants, but when we cook it at home, it's just another white carb we should cut out).
- **Batata:** Sweet potato is high in fiber and has vitamins A, B_5, B_6, C, and E, and potassium and manganese.
- **Ñame:** Yam is an excellent source of fiber and also contains vitamins A and C, iron, and some calcium.

Okay, moving along. So, we add starchy veggies to the grains section and rename it carbohydrates, now what?

I'll divide the carbs into complex and simple carbs. I know, I know, I am throwing a lot of information at you that you might never have heard before. But to understand nutrition we must be educated. And I have seven-plus years of nutrition science education that I am going to make super easy for you to understand. I would not be my full dietitian self if I didn't break this down.

Simple carbohydrates

- Simple carbohydrates are made up of one or two sugar molecules, which are quickly digested and absorbed by the body.
- Some examples of simple carbohydrates are the sugars found in fruits (fructose), table sugar (sucrose), and milk (lactose).
- Simple carbs are found in foods like candy, soda, pastries, and other sweets.

- They provide quick bursts of energy, but lead to a rapid increase in blood sugar.

Complex carbohydrates

- Complex carbohydrates are made up of multiple sugar molecules that are bonded together.
- They take longer to break down during digestion, providing a slower and more sustained release of energy.
- Examples of complex carbohydrates include whole grains (e.g., corn, quinoa, oats), legumes (e.g., beans, lentils), and starchy vegetables (e.g., potatoes, sweet potatoes).
- Complex carbs are often high in fiber, which helps with digestion, keeps you feeling full for longer, and supports overall gut health.

Basically, simple carbohydrates are like quick-burning fuel that provides a rapid burst of energy, while complex carbohydrates are the slow-burning fuel that releases energy gradually and sustains you for longer periods. We need to take in both complex and simple carbs daily. In terms of quantity, your needs are based on how much you move throughout the day, and working with your medical team can help you figure that out. For instance, someone with heart disease who is managing their blood sugar will need more complex carbs while someone running a marathon will need more simple carbs.

MAKE A QUARTER OF YOUR PLATE PROTEIN

No one really has any issues with protein; we all know we need it and it's good for us. Plant- or animal-based, you get to choose.

Protein Sources

- **Animal-based proteins:** In the Latine community, animal-based proteins are commonly consumed. These include sources such as lean meats (e.g., chicken, beef, pork), fish, eggs, and dairy products like milk, cheese, and yogurt.
- **Plant-based proteins:** Plant-based proteins are also prominent in Latine cuisine. Examples include beans (such as black beans, pinto beans, and kidney beans), lentils, chickpeas, and quinoa.

The Importance of Protein

- **Provides the essential amino acids.** Proteins are made up of building blocks called amino acids, nine types of which the body cannot produce on its own, so they're called the essential amino acids. Consuming protein-rich foods ensures an adequate intake of these essential amino acids. Animal-based proteins are considered "complete" proteins because they contain all nine essential amino acids. Most plant-based proteins are incomplete, but they can be combined strategically to supply a complete amino acid profile. I see you, arroz blanco and habichuelas (beans).
- **Builds and maintains muscles.** Proteins are essential for building, repairing, and maintaining muscle tissue.
- **Provides essential nutrients.** Proteins from various sources offer a range of essential nutrients. Animal-based proteins often provide high-quality protein along with essential vitamins and minerals such as iron, zinc, vitamin B_{12}, and calcium. Plant-based proteins offer fiber, antioxidants, and other phytonutrients that contribute to overall health and disease prevention.

Protein-rich dishes and recipes hold cultural significance in Latine cuisine. Traditional foods like grilled meats, stews with beans and meat, or plant-based dishes like beans and rice are not only flavorful but also provide nourishment while connecting individuals to their cultural heritage.

At the end of the day, it doesn't matter if you choose to get your protein from an animal or a plant. Just be sure you're getting it from a variety of sources, especially those of you on a vegan or vegetarian diet. When you follow a diet that restricts specific food groups for personal or religious reasons, it is helpful to work with a dietitian to make sure you are properly nourishing yourself. I think another reason why our foods get a bad rep is because of frying a lot, particularly when it comes to proteins, like chuletas, chicken, fish, and chicharron. Should we fry everything? No. Do we have technology now to reduce the oil but still get the fried texture? Yes. (Hello, air fryer, please sponsor me. I have four of them!)

From an anthropological perspective, we fry foods for various reasons:

- **For preservation.** Frying can serve as a method of food preservation because it removes moisture, and without moisture bacteria cannot grow. This is especially important in regions with limited access to refrigeration or where fresh ingredients may not be readily available year-round.
- **For flavor enhancement.** Frying can enhance the flavor, aroma, and texture of foods. The Maillard reaction, which occurs when high heat interacts with the amino acids and sugars in food, creates delicious flavors and browning (which you know you love). Frying can create a crispy exterior while maintaining a moist and flavorful interior, and that's the texture I love the most in foods.
- **Resource efficiency.** Frying can be an efficient cooking method, especially in areas where fuel is scarce. Frying does

require fat, which we tend to reuse a lot, saving money on oil resources because we reuse the same batch of oil so much. It allows for the efficient transfer of heat, reducing the cooking time and conserving resources.

- **Social and cultural significance.** Frying is deeply rooted in the culinary traditions and cultural practices of many societies. It can be associated with celebrations and communal gatherings. Fried foods may hold symbolic meanings, reflecting cultural identity and traditions.
- **Adaptation to local resources.** The availability of specific ingredients and cooking mediums influences culinary practices. Cultures in regions with a lot of oil-producing crops or animal fats may have historically utilized frying as a cooking method to make use of local resources. For example, cultures with access to palm oil, olive oil, or other traditional oils may have developed frying techniques as a result.
- **Practicality and convenience.** Frying is a quick and efficient way to cook foods, especially things that are small or thinly sliced. It's practical for street food vendors, allowing for speedy preparation and immediate consumption. And you know what, the fritura lady on the corner in DR is one of my favorite people to support because of sustainability—she is frying up all the parts of the animal that in my opinion would not taste good otherwise, leaving nothing to be wasted.

Instead of labeling these cooking methods as "bad," we need to recognize that people are amazing and have found ways throughout history to live and sustainably use resources. Like I said, now we have the technology that means we do not technically have to fry everything, but frying food every once in a while won't define your health.

MAKE HALF YOUR PLATE FRUITS AND VEGGIES

It is beyond me how people fear eating fruits because of the carbs and sugar they contain. Like, por qué? Who hurt you? Not fruits. We should be eating fruits and veggies, and when MyPlate was being developed, I believe the decision to make half the plate fruits and veggies was done for two reasons: 1) to increase the amount of fruits and veggies we eat, which I totally agree with. Many of my clients benefited from consuming more fruits and veggies. And 2) to fill people up with fiber and fewer calories. That, I do not agree with.

In a country where some people may not have reliable access to nutritious foods, we should not be trying to underfeed people. Instead, we should be ensuring they have access to good-quality calories, not fewer of them.

Here are some of the many reasons we should all be eating fruits and veggies:

- **Nutrient density.** Fruits and vegetables are powerhouses when it comes to nutrients. They're loaded with all the good stuff, like essential vitamins, minerals, and fiber. Think vitamin C, vitamin A, potassium, folate, and those antioxidants. These nutrients are vital for overall health and well-being, keeping us feeling good.
- **Disease prevention.** A diet rich in fruits and veggies can be very helpful in the fight against chronic diseases. We're talking about heart disease, certain cancers, and diabetes. How does it work, you ask? Well, those fruits and vegetables are packed with antioxidants, fiber, and other amazing compounds called "phytonutrients" that team up to protect our bodies by reducing the risk of inflammation and diseases, and keep us going strong.

- **Fiber and digestive health.** Fruits and vegetables come to the rescue with their fiber content. Fiber promotes healthy digestion, keeps things moving smoothly, and helps us maintain regular trips to the bathroom. Trust me, a happy gut is a happy you!
- **Hydration and fluid intake.** Now, imagine being in a Latin American country with a hot-ass climate. Hydration is key, my friends! That's where our fruits and veggies come in. Many of them are packed with water, keeping us hydrated and our fluid balance on point. So, when it's hot outside, load up on those hydrating fruits and veggies to keep yourself feeling fresh and ready to take on the day!

Fruits and vegetables are integral to Latin American foods. Traditional dishes often have a variety of colorful fruits and vegetables, like juguitos and agua frescas.

When I think of juguitos, I think of how my family makes the most delicious jugo de tamarindo. I think of how when you go to any of our countries you are greeted at breakfast with fresh-squeezed orange juice loaded with all the vitamin C you need for the day. I think of how those eight to ten ounces of juice are perfectly portioned to give you the boost you need.

Originally from Mexico and Central America, agua frescas are a delightful blend of fresh fruits, cereals, flowers, or seeds mixed with sugar and water. These beverages, with their refreshing and hydrating essences, celebrate the flavors of fruits such as watermelon, cantaloupe, and lime. Some traditional versions even incorporate unique ingredients like hibiscus flowers or chia seeds, adding to the rich tapestry of flavors.

From a nutritional standpoint, agua frescas are loaded with benefits. Being primarily fruit-based, they are natural sources of essential vitamins like vitamins C, A, and various B's. The specific fruit chosen determines the vitamin content, with all of them providing tons of benefits like bolstering immune defenses and ensuring skin health and efficient energy metabolism. Their water-based composition makes them excellent sources of hydration, and the flavorful twist they give to a hydration routine appeals to those seeking an alternative to the routine of plain water.

Beyond their hydration value, the antioxidant properties of many of the ingredients used in agua frescas, especially berries, citrus fruits, and hibiscus flowers, deserve mention. These molecules combat oxidative stress (a state in which the body has too many free radicals), potentially fending off chronic ailments. When the fruit's pulp is included in an agua fresca, the beverage also offers dietary fiber, promoting better digestion.

However, it's the customization potential of agua frescas that truly makes them stand out. Agua frescas that combine characteristic flavors not only pay homage to rich culinary traditions but also offer a harmonious blend of taste and nutrition. They are a testament to how beverages can be both indulgent and beneficial, offering a symphony of flavors while nourishing the body.

Now, imagine my surprise when the TikTok trend of "spa waters" went viral—it was nothing but a whitewashing of such an amazing cultural drink. Per usual, the framing was that these creators "discovered" agua frescas and dubbed them "spa waters" to fit their tongues, because apparently saying "agua fresca" is too hard. Many white TikTokers took to the app to discuss their newfound "spa water" flavors without discussing the drink's origin or using the proper name. When called out about it, they would say things like, *It's not that serious, it's just flavored water.* But it *is* serious because our foods get "discovered" and gentrified daily. Meanwhile, in the same breath we are told our foods are bad for us, until they save us by making it "healthier." I will say it now and

I will say it a million times over, our foods are healthy. Always have been, always will be.

DAIRY

Now dairy is off to the side in the MyPlate graphic, signifying how Americans grew up drinking a glass of milk with dinner, which we know many of us did not, but I digress. It's important to not dismiss dairy immediately just because our cultures don't drink it straight out of a glass. It still can provide you with good and complete nutrition *if* you choose to drink it.

Dairy is all three macronutrients, and I freaking love it. I love dairy because it can give me a lot of nutrition, including hydration, protein, carbs, calcium, potassium, vitamin D, and vitamin A in eight ounces. It is versatile, and my barriguita loves it. Dairy intake varies depending on ethical values, intolerances, and personal reasons.

You don't have to like it or drink it. You might even have lactose intolerance (a condition in which you have trouble digesting lactose, the sugar found in milk and other dairy products), which makes it tricky for you. Now, here's the deal: The prevalence of lactose intolerance varies across the globe by region and population.

Lactose intolerance tends to be more common in communities with a history of limited dairy consumption, like many African, Asian, and Native American groups. These folks don't make enough of an enzyme called lactase, which breaks down lactose, after being weaned. That means that digesting lactose is trickier, leading to symptoms like bloating, gas, diarrhea, and tummy discomfort.

But here's where it gets interesting: Populations in places like Europe and North America, where dairy has been a big part of the culinary scene for ages, have actually evolved to handle lactose better. They've got something called lactase persistence, which means that instead of declining after weaning, lactase production keeps going into adulthood. This genetic adaptation makes it easier for them to digest lactose and enjoy dairy products without the same panza troubles.

Globally, it's estimated that about 65 to 70 percent of people have some degree of lactose intolerance; thankfully, I am not one of those people. And for the record, the less dairy you eat, the less lactase you produce, which makes digestion of lactose-containing products like dairy difficult. Now, let's focus on different regions. East Asia takes the lead with a whopping estimated prevalence of lactose intolerance ranging from 70 to 100 percent. That's right, my friends, lactose intolerance is pretty darn common in these parts.

In African, Native American, and other Asian populations, lactose intolerance also has a strong presence, affecting approximately 50 to 80 percent of individuals. These folks have a higher chance of feeling the effects of lactose intolerance. On the other hand, people of Northern European descent tend to have lower rates of lactose intolerance, with estimates ranging from 5 to 20 percent. It seems they've got a bit more tolerance for the lactose game.

But hey, let's remember that dietary recommendations need to be flexible and consider individual needs. If you can't do dairy, no worries! There are plenty of other sources of important nutrients like calcium and vitamin D. Fortified plant-based milks, leafy greens, fortified cereals, and other calcium-rich foods can do the trick.

The bottom line is that knowing about lactose intolerance and catering to different dietary needs lets folks make informed choices about dairy consumption and helps us create inclusive recommendations.

DISMANTLING THE STEREOTYPE THAT LATINO FOODS ARE "BAD"

Now, one thing I will say forever and ever is that just because the people who created the dietary recommendations may have never stepped foot in our countries and perpetuate stereotypes (knowingly or unknowingly) does not mean our foods are not good or nutritious. Unfortunately, the truth is that although the United States is very diverse, making recommendations that are diverse is apparently hard for the people in charge. But as you'll see in this chapter, it's not that complicated to incorporate more diverse foods.

On my call with the MyPlate peeps, they told me they had been tasked with making MyPlate a household name. You know how I would do that? I'd bring in the abuelitas from across the globe and have a public health nutrition campaign that has them cooking traditional dishes, and then bring in dietitians from the community to advise them on how to make the foods as nutritious as they are delicious. This is a very important part in people being seen!

Although some efforts are being made to widen the array of foods said to be healthy by the USDA's standards makers, cultural foods are often labeled "bad." Nutrition, as I shared from my college education experience, is whitewashed. My education taught me that the reason my community was sick was because of our foods, but it failed to address the racist systems that are in place that keep our people without access to food and healthcare. It taught me that Eurocentric foods are inherently better. For instance, when you think of kale, you think that it's a highly nutritious, gold-standard vegetable for the wellness girlies, but when you think of collard greens, you probably consider it to be a lesser, not-as-popular vegetable. Why is that? Well, for one, one of these foods is associated with white elites, while the other is associated with Black communities. They are virtually the same nutritionally. I mean, I can go on and on about this. But the truth is, if dietitians and medical providers who have the knowledge about our foods aren't speaking up, nothing will change. Because perspectives across the board need to be changed, from public health to medicine to health policy, and that won't happen with us being quiet.

This is also a great time to discuss flavors, spices, and seasonings. Remember Dr. Kellogg? He believed that spicy or flavorful foods could lead to sinful thoughts and behaviors. The primary purposes of the bland diet he recommended were to promote a healthy lifestyle and to curb what he considered unhealthy desires. Today, "healthy" foods are associated with minimal seasonings and flavors, and this may be where it comes from. When our foods are demonized for being too spicy, too flavorful, this is an attempt by white elites to differentiate themselves from us.[2] And this was not just Kellogg's idea. When the Global South was colonized, Europeans gained access to sabor, and a lot of it. I know that many of us wonder why, if they had access to so many spices, is their food so bland? I know it's a running joke, but there is a reason for this. Once the monarchy and elites realized that the lower classes had access to spices, they no longer wanted anything to do with them because they needed to be "different" and "better," more "refined," and thus they created the idea of less flavorful foods.[3] Using fewer spices was cleaner, more natural, simpler. They chose to have less sabor so they wouldn't be like us. And today, when your wellness gurus want to be better, different, healthier than us, they revert back to these ideologies to separate themselves and their followers from the commoners.

The cuisine of Latin America is broad and delicious. From seafood to pastries, traditional recipes are full of flavor, memories, and energy. Because there are so many misconceptions surrounding these dishes, let's discuss some common ingredients in our dishes and their nutritional value.

Corn

Let's cut through the confusion around corn. Is it a grain, a veggie, or a fruit? Corn is a whole grain, and whole grains are considered fruits because they're the seeds of a plant. What is important to remember is that corn—like that used for our tortillas and masas—is packed with nutrition. Indigenous peoples in Mesoamerica knew this. They had this brilliant process called "nixtamalization," which involves soaking corn kernels in an alkaline solution,[4] most commonly calcium hydroxide and water, which boosts the availability of essential nutrients like niacin and calcium. A lack of niacin (vitamin B_3) in the diet causes pellagra, a systemic disease that can lead to death if left untreated, so this wasn't just a culinary technique, it was a lifesaver.

Corn is also one of the legendary "Three Sisters," alongside beans and squash. In Indigenous Latin American agriculture, these three were the ultimate #SquadGoals. They were planted together because they help each other out: Beans enrich the soil with nitrogen, corn provides a natural trellis for the beans to climb, and squash keeps the soil moist with its large leaves. This was sustainability before sustainability was even a thing! When colonizers took corn across the world but left without this crucial knowledge of nixtamalization, this caused health problems like pellagra among the colonized communities. So the next time you're biting into corn on the cob or having some good-ass masa, remember that you're not just getting a delicious bite; you're also connecting with centuries of Indigenous wisdom. This knowledge isn't just for counting nutrients; it's about respecting them.

Beans

I call beans "habichuelas," and I know many call them "frijoles." One cup of pinto beans is *loaded* with nutrition; it's going to give you fifteen grams of protein, fifteen grams of fiber, and 20 percent of your daily iron needs, as well as calcium, magnesium, and potassium. They're affordable, they're nourishing, and when you combine them with arroz, you create a nutritious and cheap meal that nourishes your body and your soul.

Have you ever stopped and wondered why the narrative on rice and beans is so skewed? On one hand, when a vegetarian or vegan chooses white rice and beans, this dish is considered nutritionally great for them because it provides all the essential amino acids. On the other hand, my mom was told by her Colombian doctor that the traditional arroz con habichuela meals that I grew up eating daily are too high in carbs. The doctor told her she has to pick one or the other, meaning that rice or beans never go together. That's because even those who are also from a nonwhite culture have been conditioned to think a certain type of food is better and healthier. Foods labeled "vegan" or "vegetarian" are considered healthier by the wellness world. Depending on who is walking into that doctor's office, the recommendation will change. It's the same dish, it's just that one person or way of eating is valued more.

Let's dive into beans. Y'all know I love talking about food history, and beans have quite the story that deserves a shout-out.

Beans are one-third of the legendary Three Sisters trio, but European colonizers once again took without understanding.

When they landed in the Americas, the colonizers were quick to grab both corn and beans and take them back home. But just like with corn, they failed to grasp the whole picture and didn't plant them together. They took the crops but left behind the wisdom that made the Three Sisters such an agricultural and nutritional powerhouse. They also missed the fact that these crops weren't just foods; together, they were a symbol of community and coexistence. Fast-forward to today, and beans are still global superstars, loaded with protein and nutrients and a key player in dishes all around the world. So the next time you enjoy an amazing bowl of rice and beans, remember you're not just eating, you're also connecting with a rich tapestry of history and culture.

Squash/Calabaza

Squash, or, as some might know it, "calabaza," is the least-hyped but still crucial member of the Three Sisters. The backbone of Indigenous agriculture in the Americas, squash is not there just to fill space; it's a nutrient powerhouse packed with vitamins A and C, fiber, and potassium, and its broad leaves make it a moisture-saving genius in the field by acting like nature's mulch to keep the soil moist.

Squash has been cultivated for thousands of years, first by Indigenous peoples in Mesoamerica before it was expropriated by Europeans and taken around the globe. Each culture that adopted squash added its own culinary flair to its preparation, but the core benefits remained the same: It's versatile and nutritious, and its nutrients play well with others. Squash complements the protein from beans and the whole grain goodness from corn, making meals not just balanced but also culturally rich.

Platanos

I grew up eating a lot of platanos (after all, I am Dominican), and as I got older, I learned that people in other countries eat them too but have different names for the dishes I love. We all have different names for dishes that are very similar, like mangu and mofongo. Platanos maduros and verdes—we all eat them, we love them, and they are so versatile. In terms of possible uses and nutrition, I would compare platanos to potatoes. They are rich in fiber; in vitamins A, C, and B$_6$; and in magnesium and potassium.

Onions and Peppers (Sofrito and Salsas)

In case you need to hear it from a dietitian, onions and peppers count as veggies too! There is a persuasive narrative that unless it's a piece of kale or broccoli, it doesn't count. The diet and wellness culture has a funny way of elevating certain foods its enthusiasts consider "super" while demonizing others. The truth is, all veggies will give you fiber, vitamins, and minerals, and there's no reason why a mommy blogger should be praised for pureeing broccoli into mac and cheese while our mamis get no credit for loading the sofrito into our foods. And, *yes,* those onions, peppers, and herbs count in our nutrient tallies. They do not disappear. They might not have the *full* amount that's recommended for the day, but it adds up. Again—sorry if I sound like a broken cantaleta—the goal is to eat a variety of foods throughout the day.

Because we all call things by different names in our separate countries, it wasn't until I became a dietitian that I realized that the molondrones or berenjena I ate when I was growing up were okra and eggplant. There are so many foods my mom cooked that I thought were bad based on the rhetoric I was hearing that turned out to have been hella nutritious all along. What I am trying to say is, if MyPlate really wants to make a change, if the USDA is really interested in making recommendations that are diverse and culturally humble, they will hire dietitians from the community who can adapt nutritional information so it aligns with Latine cultures so our people can feel seen.

THE PUSH FOR EUROCENTRIC DIETARY RECOMMENDATIONS

The "Mediterranean diet" refers to the traditional dietary habits of some of the countries bordering the Mediterranean Sea. Often celebrated for its health benefits, it's frequently discussed in wellness circles and by health professionals. But while there's no denying the nutritional merits of the Mediterranean diet, it's essential to also consider the broader context in which it is promoted. It's championed to the extent that it sidelines or even outright dismisses the significance of non-European foods, many of which are just as nutritious and culturally valuable. Take quinoa, for instance. This ancient grain, native to the Andean region, boasts numerous health benefits and has been a staple in South American diets for millennia. Yet it gained global recognition only in recent decades, while foods from European diets have been widely celebrated for much longer. It was just in the early 2000s that quinoa gained popularity due to the rise of the gluten-free eating trend; the United Nations named 2013 the International Year of Quinoa, and restaurants started jumping on the bandwagon by adding it to their menus.

Now, I know you have all heard of the Mediterranean diet and how beneficial and flavorful it is. It's all about embracing whole foods, plant-based ingredients, healthy fats, and moderate amounts of animal products. Sounds great, right? Well, here's where things get a bit complicated. Critics like me argue that cultural foods from nonwhite countries are overlooked or disparaged in comparison. Non-European foods are perceived as inferior, while European foods are upheld as the gold standard. This Eurocentric bias not only affects our perceptions of what's "good" or "bad" for us, but can also lead to the erasure of diverse culinary traditions and histories.

For instance, the Mediterranean diet emerged from the traditions of the European countries bordering the Mediterranean Sea, but it leaves out the North African and Middle Eastern countries that also border the sea and use many of the same ingredients or different ones with equivalent nutritional value. These countries have their own unique and tasty dishes, and it's problematic that the Mediterranean diet is celebrated as the gold standard while these other equally nutritious and diverse dietary traditions are overlooked or labeled as "less than."

For instance, hummus is often hailed as the perfect snack food because it's made with chickpeas and olive oil, but refried beans made with lard are viewed negatively. In reality, these are both legume-based sides that have fats in them. While people commonly assume that lard serves no purpose in cooking, it is rooted in the cultural practice and in the sustainability of using the whole animal to decrease waste.

Like shawarma, al pastor is marinated and cooked on a revolving spit, but chicken shawarma has a better reputation than chicken al pastor even though they are basically the same except for having different spices.

And while the Mediterranean diet does boast a lot of fresh fruits and veggies, we often forget that salsas and marinades are also made of veggies. Not to mention all the fresh fruit that is sold by street vendors in Latin American countries. No cuisine is better than the other; we just prepare many of the same foods in different ways.

This Eurocentric bias can lead to a marginalization of non-European cultures and their foods. It disregards the richness of African, Middle Eastern, and other non-European food traditions that have their own valuable health benefits. By putting the Mediterranean diet on a pedestal, we risk ignoring the diverse range of foods and ingredients that exist beyond its boundaries.

So it's time to recognize the racism lurking in the promotion of the Mediterranean diet. Let's shift our focus to embracing and respecting the incredible diversity of food traditions and making space for all cultures and their respective healthy eating patterns. Doing so will set us on a journey toward creating an equitable and inclusive food narrative that truly celebrates the richness of our traditions. Because all our foods are good, not just those of a particular region.

WHITE RICE VERSUS BROWN RICE

I often think about how "brown" rice is highly recommended in the Mediterranean diet. It's a whole grain. Which, yes, we want! You read above why whole grains are so important, but why are they promoting brown rice specifically?

Honestly, when I became a dietitian and started my social media accounts, I did not expect my stance on white rice to be so controversial. But here we are in a wellness world that hates white rice and consistently tries to shove brown rice down our throats in the name of health. But let me ask you a question. Do you know of any dish from the Mediterranean or anywhere in the world that, without having been healthified, uses brown rice? The answer is probably no. We have mixed dishes, we have red rice, wild rice, all different kinds of rice. But brown rice by itself is an American thing. Yes, we want those whole grains, but guess what? We can get them in so many other ways; brown rice is not the only whole grain. And quite frankly it's the least tasty one. We need to stop erasing cultural dishes in the name of "health" because we can add fiber and nutrients in many other ways.

Another fun fact that so many people do not realize is that all white rice starts as brown rice. We take the bran (brown shell) off because it makes it more digestible and tastier, but in doing this, we lose some nutrients, specifically 1 gram of fiber. That processing, which is not something to fear, changes white rice into a "processed" or "refined" food, which doesn't mean that it's unhealthy, it just means the original structure has been changed. Taking off that bran and losing that fiber and some micronutrients is not the end of the world: We can add it back twofold in the forms of the beans, veggies, and protein in the rest of your meal. People rarely eat rice alone, but if you do, there's nothing wrong with that either.

Back in the day, brown rice was a food for the peasants because only the rich could afford the labor-intensive white rice. Eventually, with modernization, it became the rice most of us eat. Then, in the early twenty-first century, nutrition and wellness people began to hyperfocus on the miniscule differences between white and brown rice, largely due to the "eat whole grains" lens. As a result, brown rice has gone from a "peasant food" to the "it girl." Funny how trends change.

Now, let's return to Eva, who embodies everything I care about when I talk about nutrition. She took a deep dive into our traditional foods, learned about their nutritional gold via my nutrition library,° and whipped up meals that were both tasty and guilt-free.

° Shout out to my Latina Nutrition Library Membership, which exists so my clients can embrace their culture and nutrition. ☺

She kept her traditions alive and saw some amazing changes, and not just in herself. She was able to educate her whole fam.

Eva's journey wasn't just about getting healthy. It was about weaving together health, family, and a big ol' dose of culture, making sure it stays real and doesn't get lost in translation. She learned to find health, manage her blood sugar, and still eat all of her Puerto Rican foods.

TLDR: You matter, your taste buds matter, your traditions matter. Your cultural foods are loaded with balanced macronutrients, micronutrients, and fibers that nourish your body. If we erase our cultural foods, we erase all the amazing meals our ancestors created out of the land they had. Through all the hardships they endured, they created meals that still nourish us and give us all the nutrition we need. And that's freaking amazing.

CHULA PRACTICE: Consider using a cultural ingredient you haven't cooked with in a while. Find a recipe or ask your relatives for theirs and prepare this dish for yourself!

PART TWO

The CHULA Method

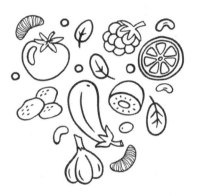

CHALLENGE THE
NEGATIVE THOUGHTS

WHEN I first started selling my services, I focused primarily on Intuitive Eating and Health at Every Size, which I still do. But I wanted to add some sazón to things, because if we as Latinas, Latine, Latinx are going to be part of a movement, we first need to feel seen by the movement. And our cultura has to be part of it. We have so much pride in our traditions, and they have to be part of why we do this. Health is important to us, as it should be. But we should not have to erase ourselves in the process.

This is why I took what I teach every day and created the CHULA Method. It is my way of adding sazón to the nutrition movement, and also helping you heal your relationship with food and your body. One day, I was on a one-on-one call with a chula (who happened to be a marketer and freaking Super Bowl producer!), and she said to me, "Why don't you create a method? I mean, what you are teaching me is so valuable and you need to put a name to it." I truly had never thought of it, but after our call, it all just fell into place for me—CHULA:

Challenge the negative thoughts
Honor your body and health
Understand your needs and body cues
Listen to your hunger and fullness
Acknowledge your emotions

For this second half of the book, we will be breaking down my CHULA Method to help you find real health and healing.

Let's begin with challenging those negative thoughts. As a woman, you no doubt contend with them *everywhere*! We have negative thoughts about our bodies, what we eat, how productive we are, even how good we are at parenting. Just about *everything* seems to be negative. But functioning in the negative is not for me, and it shouldn't be for you either. However, I'd like to clarify that I am not talking about toxic positivity, because I do not believe we can just positively think our way into happiness. But when it comes to food and our bodies, when we add in food and exercise from a positive place, it helps us feel better.

CHULA STORY: DALINA!

When I was going to Penn State for my bachelor's in nutritional sciences, I was the *only* Latina. I remember there being one Black girl and a few Asians. We were the outliers. My senior year was 2009–2010, *peak* Michelle Obama's Let's Move! campaign time. The fight against "obesity" was going strong, and as future dietitians, my classmates and I were *in* it. We were going to save everyone— at least that's what I believed. Now, there is nothing wrong with the ideas in the campaign: healthier school meals, more physical activity, healthier families, better access to affordable and healthy food, public–private partnerships promoting healthful behaviors, and childcare improvements—those are all great things to strive for. The issue with this and many similar campaigns is that the people on the ground, the ones who really need it, don't get the benefits. These ideas are too broad to actually fix the systemic issues, and unfortunately, diet culture ends up taking those healthy behaviors to the extreme.

In my classes, all we learned was how to "fix" my community, how to "fix" the food, how to "fix" the people's health, and how to make them better, basically by erasing any inch of culture they had left. I was inundated with negative thoughts about my community based on what everyone was saying. In every course, I was taught to tell people who looked like me to switch from white rice to brown because it was "better." I was taught that Latine foods are higher in fat and mostly fried and therefore should be avoided. I wrestled with what I was learning because my lessons were telling me my mami's food was bad. They were telling me that the community I grew up with was bad, that processed and fried foods were the issue. But not once did they mention how redlining prevented BIPOC communities from building generational wealth and how the Federal-Aid Highway Act of 1956 disproportionately tore down BIPOC communities by routing new highways through their neighborhoods, often leaving them in food swamps, areas where fast-food restaurants and corner stores are more prevalent than places to buy fresh fruits and vegetables. While growing up in Philadelphia, I walked those streets. I knew that those people did not have access to healthy food. And I knew something had to change; I just did not have the words for it.

I couldn't grasp at the time that just because my foods weren't being studied or showcased in my curriculum, it didn't mean they were bad. Somewhere in the back of my mind, I could hear my abuela's voice and feel her love for our traditional dishes. But in that moment, back in 2010, I genuinely believed that it was our food making my community sick—and I was going to be the one to "save" them.

Whenever I've been asked about nutrition by the media, or even when I was trying to land a book deal, the question has always been: Why do Latinas need this information? What makes your approach different from what's already out there? My response has always been the same: because, to my knowledge, no one has talked about our comida and our comunidad in a positive light.

Every single article, research paper, media clip, Instagram post, etc., that I see speaks down on our foods. You can see it regularly on TikTok. One of my most viral videos is me speaking up against a Mexican cardiologist who told her followers that eating refried beans and tortillas (along with other food staples in the Mexican diet) was the reason that Latines have higher rates of heart disease. The media is always telling us that somehow, we are going to die because of the way we eat. We will dig into all of the stats and chronic diseases in Chapter 6, but in this chapter, as we begin our journey to authentic health, you need to learn to feel compassion for yourself and to challenge the negative thoughts around your body. Then, when we aren't focused on fitting into a mold that was never meant for us, we can focus on real nutrition.

CHALLENGING BODY IMAGE IN OUR LATINE COMMUNITIES

We live in a world that values thinness, that values a certain look. It values more highly a certain hair type, a certain color of eyes, and certain features. We know that if we are "beautiful" by the standards of society, for the most part, there is safety in that. Of course, misogyny is still there—no one can outrun it—but there is safety and comfort in knowing that looking a certain way brings us benefits. Being pretty and thin allows you to glide through without comments. I know this: I was the thin one, and often the pretty one. I never got comments about my body or weight. (Now, my hair, that was a different story.) But the truth is, challenging negative thoughts about your body is hard. And I will never, ever minimize that. I will never tell you that wanting to lose weight, change your body, or be accepted is wrong. Because it's just a fact that it is easier to live in society when you fit a certain "type."

However, what I hope to do is to point out some of the main issues that I see in our communities that drive this ideal, and then you, and only you, can decide what to do with this information. You can decide to embrace the body you have now and focus on health behaviors, or you can come back to it later when you feel like you are in a better place. Whatever you decide is fine.

I am a millennial, and I would like to set a scene showing how the teenage years of people in my generation might have gone and why we feel the way we do about our bodies.

The year is 2004, you are in high school, and RBD is playing at home every day after school. Let me tell you about Anahí, the star of *Rebelde,* aka Mia Colucci, telenovela character, who impacted us viewers and how we saw ourselves in our communities. Recently, with the RBD reunion, Anahí has been vocal about the pressure she faced during that time to look a certain way and how it led to her developing an eating disorder. She's done a few candid interviews about how she was bullied on live TV by superfamous hosts and how it affected her. It affected her, and it also affected us.

They pushed her to be thin, to have blond hair, to speak English to seem cool, to talk like a stereotypical valley girl. We all wanted to be her, to not be the girls with the brown hair. This can plant the seeds of negative thoughts about our bodies. We were conditioned to want the flat stomach for wearing low-rise jeans, the "not too big, not too small" butt to fit the clothing, the "not too big, not too small" boobs for wearing a button-down shirt—basically an impossible standard that no one can achieve. Or if they can, they have to struggle to stay there and maintain it.

But before we discuss challenging thoughts around body image, we need to set some facts straight about the Latino community and its anti-Black beliefs. If me saying these words upsets you, makes you angry, makes you want to email me or DM me to tell me how wrong I am and ask how the heck I can sit here and say that our community is racist, then I need you to take a deep breath, journal those feelings, and do a simple Google search. The internet is free and you can get the history lessons there, or better yet, invest in Black educators who are doing the work of trying to end our culture's anti-Black bias.

If you have heard the term "mejorar la raza"—"better the race"—you cannot deny the anti-Blackness in our community that stems from colonization. That colonization led the populations of many of our Latin American countries to idolize the European ideal because there was a time when marrying someone with lighter skin to move up in the caste system was the main goal in communities in every damn country. The idolization of European features encourages diet culture and the development of eating disorders in our community.

Something else that has just as large an impact on our perception of ourselves and stems from within the Latine community is telenovelas. When I was growing up, after school you could always find me watching the novelas in the living room as my mom cooked dinner and I was supposed to be doing homework. I have vivid memories of watching *Agujetas de color de rosa,* partly because I couldn't look away from the drama unfolding on the screen and partly because I was an ice-skater at that time (which didn't last very long).

Novelas have a special place in my heart, but I also recognize that they have done a lot of damage to how we view ourselves and our bodies through underrepresentation and tokenism, colorism, self-perception, and stereotyping.

Indigenous and Black actresses are historically underrepresented in leading roles in novelas. I tried to think of one novela, just one, that I could remember from when I was growing up that had a Black or Indigenous protagonista. I googled, and you guessed it, *zero*. I did, however, come across an article in *Hispanic Executive*— "Hisplaining: Why Most Mexican Telenovela Stars Are Güeros,"[1] in which author Laura Martinez explains:

> Growing up in Mexico City, watching telenovelas, and being exposed to a constant bombardment of TV commercials, I was convinced that most Mexicans were blue-eyed blonds. . . . [The] overrepresentation of white people in my country was a consequence of a harsh reality . . . colorism exists and is not limited to my birth country.

And I can 100 percent say this is also true in the Dominican Republic. There is more diversity on locally produced TV shows, but the commercials? I was always so confused. How could these blondes be selling us this stuff? Truly mind-boggling, but not surprising. The underrepresentation plus the colorism made many of us feel like we were not enough. I never saw anyone who looked like me. No one with curly hair, and honestly no one with my accent, unless I was in DR watching a local show. The mainstream media looked a lot like America, and I am not talking about Ferrera.

The cultural obsession with the Miss Universe contest further promotes colorism. Many of the contestants are very fair-skinned even when their country of origin is comprised of mostly dark people, reinforcing the idea that lighter skin is more beautiful.

By watching these shows and commercials all the time, we were told who we should want to be. We wanted to be blond, tall, and skinny because let's be honest, body diversity was not a thing then, and still is not now. Those of us who did not fit the mold had to try to achieve whiteness in other ways, and that often meant straightening our hair daily and dyeing it a lighter color.

On the rare occasions when we are represented in the media, the characters are stereotypes such as poor, uneducated maids. Never are we in the main storyline unless we are getting smacked around by the patrón.

Take one of the most popular novelas of all times as a case study: *Yo soy Betty, la fea*, or as many Americans know it, *Ugly Betty*.

Betty, la fea was a novela I am pretty sure we all saw even if it was the Colombian version or the American version: the tale of an ugly duckling who turns beautiful and gets her Prince Charming, such a happy ending. But the issue with this trope and eternal storyline is that it says that women, trans people, nonbinary folks, and others are not worthy until they fit society's idea of beauty. It's always "Oh, she is so smart, so competent, but if she was pretty, she could really succeed." And inevitably, Betty does. She goes full supermodel and gets the man and the company.

And we think it's such a beautiful story. But why? We are literally teaching girls that they are worthy only if they fit conventional European beauty standards. Betty had to become skinnier before she could be worthy. She straightened her hair, got rid of her glasses, and changed the way she spoke, all to be more "professional."*

---

* Woo, we could have a whole-ass conversation about respectability politics, but I would just ask you to go read Chrissy King's book, *The Body Liberation Project*. She will explain it better than I ever could.

It's just really sad that our cultural obsession with whiteness and thinness is embedded into our everyday lives by the media and our families.

I remember spending late nights as a kid when I used to sleep over at my tía's house watching my prima order all the stuff from the infomercials. Classic 1990s stuff. One weekend, she bought a cast faja (girdle) that was meant to give you a Thalia waist, but we all knew that was probably not possible, since the rumor was that Thalia had had ribs taken out in order to get that slim figure (yes, I know, wild!). Nonetheless, that didn't stop this prima from ordering it, and I am pretty sure she had to return it when it came in because my tía was not having it. To this day, we still crack up at all the infomercial crap she bought.

And although I think of these memories generally fondly because I was always having a good time with my prima, years later, I see more clearly how all these moments of desiring to be skinnier or to look like a certain novela star impacted our perceptions of ourselves.

The fat-shaming and discrimination doesn't just come from TV and other media, it also comes from families. I had a video go viral in which I stitched Eva Longoria saying in a podcast interview that her nickname growing up was the prieta fea, the ugly black one. Now, we all know that nicknames like these are the norm. Whether its gorda, flaca, fea, linda, prieta, rubia, guera—they all have a physical connotation to them. And usually not a good one. We belittle our children with these nicknames, which then become their identities, often harmful ones. Ones that lead them to wanting to fit in, to no longer being gorda, to no longer being fea. And this leads to mental health issues and disordered eating habits to try to fit in. Hence the name of the novela, *Yo soy Betty, la fea.* She was fea until she fit the conventional beauty standards. And although she did it while still being herself, we know that that is not what women and girls learned from this show.

We can often pinpoint the development of our eating disorder or disordered eating back to these moments when we were at impressionable ages. I often think about quinceañera parties, for coming of age, and how diet culture is steeped into these traditions. I can tell you that most of the chulas I work with started dieting for their quinces because they needed to fit into the dress. So many went on to use diet pills, extremely low-calorie diets, and even surgeries to meet the expectations, most with the approval of their mamis.

I once posted about quinces in my stories and so many of you messaged me. I vividly remember one message in which someone told me that her mom got prescription diet pills for her to make sure she did not gain weight after her dress was altered. I want you to let that sink in: A mother purchased diet pills for her daughter so that the fourteen-year-old would not gain weight before a party. And I know that you know that this is not an anomaly.

I thankfully did not want a quinceañera because I was in so many of them that by the time it was my turn, I was like, *Hell to the no*. But this is a rite of passage for our community, and for many, this is where disordered eating begins because this is the first time your body will be placed on display for *everyone* to see, and it has to be perfect. And not to sound like a broken cantaleta here, but what is perfect? Thinness. Now, the term "almond mom" doesn't feel right here, but "ensalada mami" might.

What I have learned from chulas' stories without a shadow of a doubt is that this generational trauma needs to end. Our kids and the generations behind them deserve to live in a world where they are not judged by their appearance.

FINDING NEUTRALITY
How to Find Neutrality with Your Body and Your Weight

Challenging the ideas about weight is hard, and I always say that if anyone tells you they don't have ideas about changing their body in some way, shape, or form, they are probably lying. We live in a society that values looks, and we all want to be accepted, and we all think about it. The difference is that some act on it, and some don't. I always ask the chulas who work with me, "What is your intention?" Intention is everything. We can want to lose weight, we can want to change our body, we all have negative thoughts, but will we do it? Is it your intention to go back to diets and change your body? Or is it your intention to just talk it out and let it go?

You get to choose your course of action. We talked about yo-yo dieting in Chapter 2, but I want to discuss weight stability here. I always say, "I want you to find weight stability." I want to remind you of why weight cycling, also known as yo-yo dieting, is so detrimental for our health. For one, it negatively impacts our metabolism and worsens insulin resistance and inflammation, all of which puts us at risk for, you guessed it, diabetes and heart disease. In a study published in the *Journal of Epidemiology and Community Health*,[2] researchers found that when they compared females with stable weight to weight cyclers, those who had experienced weight cycling had worse lipid values and insulin resistance. They found that even those of "normal" weight who had been through multiple periods of weight cycling still had lower high-density lipoprotein (HDL, the good cholesterol) and elevated lipid levels.

This tells us that even if you are "fat," if your weight is stable, you are likely to have better lab work than those of "normal" weight whose weight has repeatedly fluctuated. This is why I focus on finding weight stability. To me, it is where you just are, where your weight fluctuates within normal parameters. For instance, in those who menstruate, hormonal changes can cause weight changes throughout the month; that is normal. Weight stability means no huge fluctuations of losing twenty pounds and then gaining forty pounds every three months—that is weight cycling. Weight stability is you being able to enjoy life, eat without fear, and go out and enjoy every day, understanding that your energy needs vary daily and so your food intake will too. It is learning to connect with and understand your needs and cues. It's literally *Eat Pray Love*, without a side of fatphobia.

Impacts of Weight Cycling
INFLAMMATION AND STRESS

Your gravitational pull on this Earth does not define your worth or health. We need to discuss the inflammation caused by weight cycling and how this increases the risks for disease and mortality. And no, I am not talking about the inflammation the wellness girlies are trying to help you fix. I am talking about the chronic inflammation that happens in the body due to stress and cortisol release and the constant destabilization of the body and metabolism that comes with dieting and weight cycling.

Weight cycling triggers stress in the cells in the entire body. It also alters your gut microbiota. All those good bacteria we want in our guts to help us digest food and create our brain hormones get disrupted during weight cycling, leading to an inflammatory response. This also triggers the immune system to perceive the rapid weight loss as a stressor and initiate inflammatory signals. The constant weight cycling (because it doesn't happen just once) then leads to chronic inflammation. So, in a weird (well, not actually weird because this is science) turn of events, the diets that the girlies are selling you to reduce inflammation are actually causing the inflammation.

HORMONAL DISRUPTIONS

We cannot talk about inflammation without talking about hormone disruptions, especially for menstruating people. This happens via various mechanisms, and it has to do with the body trying to keep up with the rapid and repeated weight fluctuations. We see it with our hormones that regulate hunger and fullness. Those hormones are leptin and ghrelin. When you start to lose weight rapidly, your leptin level begins to decrease; this is the body's way to signal the brain to eat more. Your body is wired to survive, so it sees this weight loss as a sign that something is wrong. Your production of ghrelin then increases; this is your body increasing your hunger, asking you to eat more. When diet culture tells you to use willpower, it literally misses the fact that your body will do anything to keep you safe to ensure survival.

For many in the Latine community, the idea of getting diabetes is a big stressor, and we are told that we have a higher incidence of becoming diabetic, which I'll discuss more when we talk about social determinants of health. But as far as weight cycling goes, it affects how well your cells respond to insulin, causing insulin resistance. Insulin is the hormone that helps us regulate our blood sugar by helping the sugar obtained from food get into the body's cells for energy. Insulin resistance can be due to an increase in cortisol, the stress hormone. When your body is stressed, it releases more cortisol, which causes more inflammation and metabolic dysfunction, like what you see in insulin resistance.

Reproductive hormones are also affected by weight cycling. This yo-yoing disturbs estrogen and progesterone levels, which can lead to menstrual cycle issues or the complete loss of menstruation. If we are not eating enough or if we don't have enough fat to produce hormones, one of the first things our body stops doing is producing a menstrual cycle. Why would your body do extra work? You do not need to menstruate to live, so this is one of the ways it can reduce energy expenditure. Yo-yoing also can lead to changes in thyroid hormones, such as decreasing T3 levels and slowing down your metabolism. All these hormonal disruptions make it difficult for you to sustain weight loss and also wreak havoc on your body in the process.

THE IMPORTANCE OF SUSTAINABILITY

As opposed to weight cycling, staying at a stable weight, eating enough, eating a variety of foods, exercising, and following healthy behaviors lead to better health outcomes that are actually sustainable. And trust me, I know how difficult this must be to read, to realize that what you thought was "healthy" was actually causing all the issues that you were trying to prevent in the first place. This is why diet culture is so insidious and why I say it cannot steal healthy behaviors, because you can work on those without causing ongoing stress to your body. However, in order to achieve this, those of you with weight loss as your only goal need to put it on the back burner because if that is the only goal you have, you will never keep up with healthy behaviors: The minute that weight loss doesn't happen, you will spiral and begin unhealthy habits again. And again, I will never judge you. I will always hold space for all those feelings, but I will also always urge you toward creating healthy habits.

I know many of you will ask, *But how do I get there? How do I get to the point where I won't want to lose weight? Or where I will not place any value on the number on the scale?* The answer is, there is no answer. There is no destination. You will probably never get to that point. Because diet culture is everywhere and we are human and you will inevitably have those thoughts, you will have bad days, *you will fuck up*. No one, and nothing, is perfect. So the goal is to be compassionate, to know you always have the choice to pick up those healthy habits, and to work on those healthy behaviors, because remember, weight is not a behavior.

FINDING NEUTRALITY WITH FOOD DECISIONS

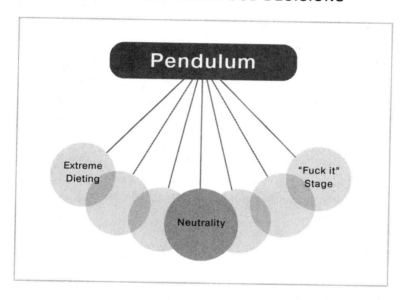

In my humble-ass opinion, finding neutrality is the goal not just with our bodies, but also with our eating habits. Being able to make a decision based on your health, taste buds, and needs at any given moment is what it's all about. I often describe this as a pendulum. We always want it swinging in the middle ever so slightly, not to the extreme ends. At one end, you have extreme dieting; at the other end, you have the "fuck it" stage.

Extreme dieting is what diet culture pushes—strict rules, restrictions, and impossible standards that are hard to maintain.

When you can't keep up with these demands, it's easy to swing to the other extreme. You might find yourself thinking, "Eff this, I'll eat whatever I want, whenever I want!" This can sometimes be mistaken for Intuitive Eating, especially after years of dieting. But this all-or-nothing approach doesn't feel good either. Without intention or awareness of your body's hunger cues, it can negatively affect your health. The goal—both your goal and my goal as your dietitian—is to help you reconnect with your cuerpo and learn how to truly listen to it.

You should aim to be in that neutral middle section of the pendulum. You'll learn to listen to your body, you'll rely on that connection to your routines and habits, and you'll realize that even though life can have bouts of stress and of calmness, you'll still be able to go with the flow (although this can be hard for my type A girlies).

Now that we've learned how to challenge negative thoughts regarding our bodies, we also need to ensure that we can challenge any negative thoughts we harbor about our food.

Challenging Negative Thoughts About Food Through Positive Nutrition

Now, let's talk about food and nutrition, my jam. I always say to my lovely chulas: Every day is a chance to add a sprinkle of good to your plate. Every meal is a new beginning. Forget taking away; let's add. That's what I call "positive nutrition." In a world where there's so much noise about what not to eat, I'm here to say, "Let's nourish." Sure, there are trends that look cool on the 'gram, but they might not vibe with how I see nutrition.

The internet is full of fearmongering about food—eating rice, bread, or fruit is suddenly a death sentence. What should we even eat, then? It's essential to challenge these negative thoughts, especially when they bad-mouth our cultural dishes. Foods that the global majority eats—white rice, different proteins, fruits, and veggies—are often overlooked in American nutritional guidelines. Yet, our ancestors thrived on these foods, and people in many other countries exhibit better health outcomes. This isn't just about nutrition; it's about the stress induced by constant food anxiety and access to food. Stressing about fats or carbs all day harms our health more than any food ever could. So, let's think critically and positively about what we eat, and honor our diverse cuisines instead of fearing them.

We are going to challenge the thoughts that these foods aren't good for us by looking at the positive nutrition in them.

First, let's reframe. You can make decisions about food that feel good! If you can think about how you can add foods or what will make them taste good, you're doing okay! You haven't fucked up! Food is always giving us energy and nutrition, and every day is different. You may have some more meal-structured days, while on others you do more grazing. For some examples, let's look at a couple of meals.

Morning: Let's say you want a donut. You probably think, *Ew, why would I want this? It's pure sugar and fat!* But we can reframe this thought by *adding* fruit for fiber, and an egg for protein, fat, and a savory taste. In doing that, you just completed an entire meal! You get to eat something you were craving *and* you can feel good about the nutrition you added to it.

Afternoon: This is a meal many of my chulas will skip or wait until two or three P.M. to eat. Maybe you have just coffee in the morning and then finally eat at two P.M. You get frustrated by being so busy that you can't even imagine pausing to eat. This leads you to have negative thoughts about the way you eat, especially if you end up hitting the vending machine for a Snickers bar or get fast food on the way home.

LET'S LEARN TO be in tune with our schedules and needs (more on this in Chapter 7) by setting a reminder to eat something, even if it's something small, for lunch. Instead of thinking you're a bad person, recognize that you are a person who lives in a world that overworks us. You're doing the best you can with what you have, and there shouldn't be any shame in that. Instead of feeling shame and guilt, focus on compassion. With everyone working so much, we will never have perfect eating.

What you can do is remind yourself that you can plan ahead, bring snacks, fill a work mini fridge, and carve out at least a little time for food. I call this the "something is better than nothing" mentality.

EVERY MEAL IS A NEW BEGINNING

I want you to focus on what you can *add* to your day, not what you can take away. You can always choose to add color to the meal in the form of a fruit or a veggie.

Having arroz blanco? Let's add fiber; you can do that with aguacates, beans, lentils, or salsa. If you're eating tacos, chula, you already have it all!—corn tortillas (a whole grain), your protein of choice, and then the cebollitas, remolachas (beets), the herbs, the salsas. And you can even add pineapple and mango. Eating avena? Add fruit, add seeds. It does not have to be all or nothing; we can add nutrition to everything we eat. And it can be authentic too.

Next, add some flavor. Always ask yourself, *What would taste good in this dish?* And no, adding kale to pollo guisado will not work. Kale is not a traditional ingredient, and in my humble opinion it does not taste right in this particular dish. If you want kale, eat it in a dish that it belongs in and will taste good in.

But you know what would taste good in that pollo guisado? Some cebolla, zanahorias, apio, some pimiento. All are veggies that add so much flavor and nutrition to that guisado. Think about the sofritos and salsas we are adding. You can add texture in the form of raw peppers and onions, jicama, zanahorias. You can add crunch with pepitas, nuts, and chili crisps. And you can add depth and temperature with cold crema or heat with spicy salsas or chilies. All of this helps us enjoy food. And the more we enjoy it, the better we digest, and the more nutrients we get.

See the difference? See how finding the positive to reframe and adding nutrition—instead of saying, *Fuck it, I ate the donut and now I suck, the day sucks, I screwed it up, might as well just send this day to hell and eat like shit* (I know you all do this)—make a difference? Because if you treat every day and every meal as a new beginning, you will see that at every meal you will probably add something. And guess what? If you don't, then you don't. On to the next meal! This way, you create a normal life, not one where you are swinging from a pendulum of bingeing on donuts to eating only salads. And that's how you challenge those negative thoughts around food. One meal and one day at a time.

TLDR: Ideally, what we want to do every day is think about where these negative thoughts are coming from, because if they're causing you stress, chula, they're not the move. Let's focus on challenging the thoughts that creep up and realizing that a lot of the "rules" and "ideologies" were not created with people who look like us in mind. Let's find neutrality with our body images by dissecting where these harmful thought patterns stem from. Challenge the thoughts of perfectionism, colorism, and the thin ideal and focus instead on the positive nutrition of all foods, especially cultural foods.

CHULA PRACTICE: Identify a recurring negative thought you have about your food choices or body. E.g., *I cannot eat a carb after six P.M.*, or *I need to lose x amount of weight before I wear the crop top.* Investigate this thought: where did it come from? Challenge it. Interrogate it. Do you really believe this or were you taught this?

6

HONOR YOUR BODY
AND HEALTH

Chula Story: Gloria

WHEN I met Gloria, she was a forty-year-old female Philadelphia City worker making $12.50 per hour. It was her first steady job in years, and for the first time in her life, she had medical insurance, which is why she ended up in my office. For most of her adult life she was only able to work part-time jobs, with no medical or dental care coverage. Her kids always had medical insurance via government assistance, but she was too proud to apply for benefits, and most of the time she didn't even qualify for it because she made "too much money." (Let that sink in.) Due to this, she had very poor dental health and diabetes. She made an appointment with me after her doctor told her she needed to get her blood sugar under control. She barely spoke English and had never been to a dietitian. She told me that she expected me to tell her to stop eating her Dominican foods and that she semi-expected never to come back to see me again.

During our first appointment, we discussed her eating habits. One of my first questions was "Can you chew?" I don't think any medical provider had ever asked her that, and she just looked at me with a ton of shame. She could not. Years of no dental benefits and years of uncontrolled blood sugar had done a number on her teeth. She shared with me that eating was really tough, so she opted for purees and soups when she had the chance to cook.

During that appointment, my sole purpose was to help her get a dental appointment. We could not focus on nutrition if she could not even chew to eat.

HEALTHCARE IN THE UNITED STATES IS COMPLICATED

In a perfect world, we would all have access to the same things. Same food, same healthcare, same housing, same education. We would all be equals. I often think about how amazing it would be if food was available to all. If everyone had access to safe housing and we all had good-quality healthcare. If medical professionals were not overworked. If kids were not hungry. If there was universal childcare, and paid parental leave. If this was the case, we could discuss health from a different place, from a place of getting to the root of an issue. I think people would be a lot happier (except for the racism and fatphobia, which are all over the world). Most European countries have universal access to healthcare, and health is better for those who live in countries that offer this.

Here in the United States, it's literally a tale of the haves and the have-nots—those who have access and those who don't. In this stage of capitalism in the United States, we see that labor and production are more important than people because even people who work are being paid pennies and denied healthcare by their own jobs. Their hours get cut so their employer doesn't have to offer health insurance, and their stress level is always high.

I live in the state of Pennsylvania, and at the time when I am writing this book, the minimum wage is $7.25. That means that a person working a full-time job at that wage—forty hours a week, for fifty-two weeks out of the year—is making $15,080 per year before taxes. *Per fucking year.* Bringing that minimum wage to $15 would mean before taxes a person would make $31,200. Now, I know that in this damn economy, that is not enough for a single person to survive on. *Period.* This country's disdain for paying fast-food workers $15 per hour because other professionals make $20 per hour and do a "real job" instead goes to show how individualism rules. The fact that people want others to suffer because they've suffered is beyond me. There are whole books that discuss this. I highly recommend *Hood Feminism* by Mikki Kendall.

FOOD ACCESS

Even people working full-time jobs have trouble accessing food and healthcare. I have had so many chulas tell me that they drive to Mexico for fresh fruits and veggies because in their border towns in Texas, it is so hard to find good-quality food. In most countries, most people go to open-air markets, butchers, and specialty stores. Everyone is brushing shoulders no matter what their class, and everyone has access to those foods. Yes, there are "supermarkets," but many countries still have specialty stores that people go to for individual items. This allows opportunities for connection, the ability to have a more personal experience when shopping, and often the purchasing of higher-quality, local foods. In the United States, that is not the case because of redlining.

Redlining is a discriminatory practice that originated in the United States in the 1930s. Financial and insurance companies and institutions would literally draw a red line on a map around neighborhoods they deemed "high risk" for loan defaults. These so-called high-risk areas were often predominantly populated by people of color, particularly Black Americans. The practice resulted in systemic disinvestment in these communities, making it difficult for residents to buy homes, start businesses, or access essential services. While explicit redlining is now illegal due to civil rights laws, the long-lasting impact of this systemic discrimination still perpetuates economic and social inequities today. Because of these practices, most BIPOC communities now do not have supermarkets because they aren't deemed profitable in these neighborhoods. These practices have really hurt BIPOC communities in more ways than we can imagine, which sets us up for our discussion of the social determinants of health.

SOCIAL DETERMINANTS OF HEALTH

The environments in which individuals are born and raised, learn, work, play, worship, and grow old influence a wide array of their health outcomes, functioning, risks, and overall quality of life.[1] These environmental circumstances are called "social determinants of health" (SDoH), and go beyond the individual's choices and genetic predispositions to include social, economic, and political factors that together contribute to health outcomes. For example, someone living in a low-income neighborhood with limited access to fresh, healthy foods, a high-quality education, and safe spaces for physical activity is more likely to experience poor health outcomes compared to someone with abundant access to these resources.

For me and my everyday practice as a Latina registered dietitian working in our communidad and also hoping to change the narratives around our communities, it is imperative that we discuss SDoH.

When we talk about health, we need to be talking about these

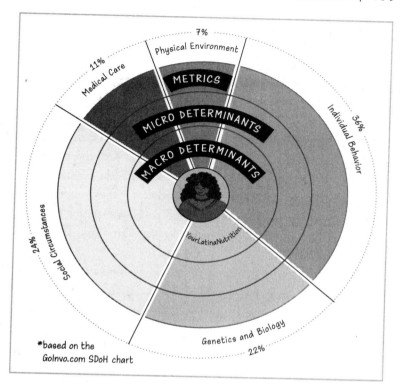

7%

Physical Environment

11%

Medical Care

METRICS

MICRO DETERMINANTS

MACRO DETERMINANTS

36%

Individual Behavior

24%

Social Circumstances

YourLatinaNutrition

Genetics and Biology

22%

*based on the
GoInvo.com SDoH chart

determinants, because only 36 percent of this chart is individual behavior (food, exercise, sleep), which is such a small percentage when you look at everything else. However, it's the part our medical system and diet culture put the most emphasis on, and I am here to challenge that. Let's discuss each piece of the pie chart.

Individual Behavior, 36 Percent:
Food, Exercise, and Sleep

If we look at the chart above, about 36 percent[2] of your health comes from eating habits, physical activity, and sleep. These are somewhat in our control. I say "somewhat" because depending on where you live and where you work, this might not be very much in your control.

Food is something that we as adults have control over for the most part. I think it's important to discuss food choices here, as in how damn stressful it is for many of us to pick what to eat! This is because society has created such a culture around food where it feels like we are damned if we eat too healthy and damned if we eat fast food. There is no nuance or gray area. And therefore, we are constantly stressing. Many people also lack basic cooking skills, and that is not something to be ashamed of. Or they might not be sure of how to create a well-balanced meal. Whatever the case may be, food is stressful, and when you are stressed, this is not good for your health!

Exercise, oh exercise. Again, we can go to the extremes on this one. Either we don't move at all *or* we overdo it. I think the one common thing when it comes to diet culture is extremeness. There is no middle ground. The "no days off" and the "go hard or go home" narratives can be very discouraging. According to the Centers for Disease Control and Prevention (CDC), there are many benefits to exercising: better mental and physical health, a reduced risk of disease, increased muscle and bone density, reduced risk for chronic diseases, and weight stability. Focusing on stability rather than weight loss encourages long-term positive behaviors; it helps us avoid the pitfalls of restriction and discouragement that often come when we don't see immediate changes in the numbers. By prioritizing stability, we can maintain a healthier, more balanced lifestyle that emphasizes the positive side of well-being rather than fixating on "loss."

Now, overexercising can have the opposite effect. According to the NIH's National Library of Medicine, overexercising can lead to feeling tired, being depressed, having mood swings and irritability, having trouble sleeping, increased numbers of injuries, experiencing anxiety, and getting more colds, just to name a few. This is why creating a healthy relationship with exercise and rest is important. We as humans are not meant to be sedentary. But also, our bodies aren't meant to go to these extremes (but I will let the exercise experts take that topic on!).

Sleep is also part of this 36 percent, and getting an adequate amount of it honestly can be super tough if you work a graveyard shift or have insomnia, or have a newborn, or are taking care of a family member. There are so many reasons why sleep can be difficult to get, and it's very important that we have self-compassion and seek help when needed.

Research shows that consistent lack of sleep is linked to higher risks of cardiovascular disease, diabetes, and hypertension. This is why it is important to find ways to make sleep—high-quality sleep—a regular part of your health routine.

Social Circumstances, 24 Percent

Next up is social circumstances, which makes up 24 percent of your health and includes your relationships in your community (social cohesion), civic participation (voting, volunteering, participating in community activities), discrimination, and incarceration.

It also takes into account:

- Racism, discrimination, language barriers, immigration status, sexual orientation, and exposure to violence
- Education, job opportunities, and income
- Access to nutritious foods and physical activity opportunities
- Polluted air and water
- Language and literacy skills

Let's look at this through the lens of immigration. Whether you are first generation or second generation, or migrated here yourself, you more than likely have been affected by a lot of this. Most people who migrate to this country deal with a language barrier, which in turn can affect educational and job opportunities. Immigrants usually move into communities that are populated largely by other immigrants, which tend to have poorer access to nutritious foods, safe sidewalks, and clean air and water due to redlining.

It's difficult to focus on "eating healthy" and exercising when you are literally fighting for your life. As mentioned before, when you have to work two or three part-time jobs to make ends meet and none of them provide you with health insurance, health is no longer something you can just "work hard for."

When you are just trying to survive, health isn't something that's top of mind. And that trauma is then passed on to members of the next generation—even the ones who have gotten out of the neighborhood—who are still struggling to understand how to take care of their needs. We saw only struggle and hustle growing up. We didn't learn to see or honor our needs, and as a result, we are still stuck in a scarcity mentality around food. It is quite the vicious cycle.

When you cannot meet your needs because doing so is simply so out of reach, whether it's paying the bills, having enough money for food, or lacking health insurance that allows you to go to a doctor's appointment, you aren't able to honor your body and health. This creates stress, which brings us to how diabetes affects the Latine community on a larger scale than other ethnicities.

Stress can have a huge impact on your blood sugar level, contributing to developing type 2 diabetes in those who are at risk or making it harder to control it. Considering what we've just discussed, we might have some genetic predisposition for diabetes, but it's known that once we get to the United States, our risk increases due to difficult SDoH.

Let's define a few terms you need to know related to blood sugar control.

- **Diabetes mellitus:** Diabetes is a condition in which your body has trouble controlling the amount of sugar, specifically glucose, in your blood. Normally, a hormone called insulin, which is produced by the pancreas, keeps your blood sugar level balanced. But if you have diabetes, your body either doesn't make enough insulin or can't use it properly, leading to too much sugar in the blood. This can cause various problems over time, like tiredness, thirst, and even damage to organs like your eyes and kidneys. Uncontrolled diabetes damages the vascular system.

  Think of your body as a car that runs on gasoline. In this example, the gasoline is the sugar in your food, and your body needs it to keep going. As we have talked about in a few chapters, sugar, aka glucose, is the body's preferred and primary source of energy. Now, to get the gasoline into the car's engine, you need a special tool or key. This tool is insulin.

- **Insulin resistance:** Imagine that one day, the lock you insert the key into is rusty. You can still put the key in, but it's hard to turn and doesn't work well. This is what's called "insulin resistance": You have insulin, but it's not doing its job well, so the sugar (the "gasoline") can't get into the cells (the "engine") to give you energy. The sugar builds up in your blood instead.

- **Diabetes:** Now, if this problem worsens and enough sugar can't get into your cells, you develop diabetes. Having too much sugar in your blood is dangerous because it can make you sick over time, affecting your heart, eyes, and kidneys, among other things.

- **Hemoglobin A1c:** This is the name of a protein produced when you metabolize sugar, as well as the name of a test that shows how well your blood sugar was controlled over the previous two to three months. Sugar left in the bloodstream because of faulty metabolism accumulates around the hemoglobin in red blood cells and is measured to see how well insulin—and therefore blood sugar control—is working.
- **Heart disease:** When diabetes is not controlled, it puts us at risk for heart disease. Because diabetes affects blood flow and vascular health (think veins, blood pressure, cholesterol), heart disease can develop as a result. "Heart disease" is a general term for issues affecting the heart's ability to circulate blood properly. This can include problems with blood flow, like blocked arteries, or issues with the heart's valves not opening and closing as they should.

Now that you have a better understanding of these conditions, let's discuss how the constant stress associated with SDoH can lead to a higher prevalence of disease.

HORMONAL RESPONSES TO CHRONIC STRESS

- **Cortisol and adrenaline release:** Experiencing stress releases hormones such as cortisol and adrenaline. These hormones prepare the body for a "fight or flight" response by releasing stored glucose and fat to supply immediate energy. While this is beneficial in the short term, chronic stress keeps these hormone levels high for extended periods, leading to elevated blood sugar and cholesterol.
- **Insulin resistance:** Persistently elevated cortisol levels make the body less sensitive to insulin, so the pancreas produces more of it to keep your blood sugar in check. But when your cells are less sensitive to insulin, they can't pull glucose from

your blood efficiently, and over time, this can develop into insulin resistance, which, as we now know, can lead to diabetes.

BEHAVIORAL FACTORS OF STRESS

- **Poor and erratic eating habits:** Stress often leads people to skip meals or to ignore their hunger. It can also mean not planning ahead and having to eat on the fly. It's very stressful for the body when you skip meals, which raises the cortisol level. And stressing about every damn thing you are going to eat and irregular eating that leads to bingeing also negatively affect the body.
- **Lack of exercise:** The demands of a stressful life can make it challenging to maintain a regular exercise routine, which is crucial for blood sugar control.
- **Impaired sleep:** Stress often affects sleep quality and quantity, and poor sleep can, in turn, contribute to poor blood sugar control.

COMPLICATIONS

- **Exacerbates existing conditions:** If you already have diabetes, stress can make it more difficult to manage, potentially leading to more frequent episodes of hyperglycemia (high blood sugar) or hypoglycemia (low blood sugar).
- **Chronic conditions:** Long-term stress along with poor blood sugar control can contribute to the development of diabetes-related complications such as heart disease, kidney disease, and nerve damage.

The stats are not great for cardiovascular disease either, with 42 percent of Hispanic women and 52 percent of men affected by it,[3] and everything discussed above also affects your heart. Stress-related releases of cortisol and other stress hormones can cause the following bodily responses.

- **The fight-or-flight response:** When you're stressed, your body goes into fight-or-flight mode: Your heart beats faster and your blood pressure goes up. If this happens often because of chronic stress, it can wear out your heart and blood vessels over time.
- **Inflammation:** Stress triggers the release of proteins and hormones that cause inflammation. Inflammation is a natural defense mechanism that keeps you safe from invading bacteria, viruses, and other bad things, but too much of it can damage your blood vessels and lead to plaque buildup, increasing the risk of heart disease.

From daily microaggressions to barely making enough income to provide food for your family, the discrimination and poverty that Latine communities have to deal with on a regular basis can cause a high level of chronic stress. It is no wonder that minority populations have a disproportionately higher rate of diabetes compared to their white counterparts.

Genetics and Biology, 22 Percent

Genetics is what it is, right? Basically, you are born with the genes you're given, and as a consequence you are predisposed to developing certain issues. We cannot change these genes, but we can certainly try to live the healthiest life possible to keep genetic risk factors at bay. So we try to eat healthy, we try to exercise, we try to get enough sleep. While there is emerging research showing that stress can alter DNA methylation and trigger genetic diseases like cardiovascular disease (CVD), this isn't being talked about enough.

Recent studies highlight how stress, especially chronic or early-life stress, can change gene expression and increase the risk for these conditions, but the research is still inconsistent and not widely discussed, leaving a gap in understanding the true impact of stress on our health.[4]

We are sold the lie that we will somehow never get sick if we just do the "right thing." So we spend years of our lives yo-yo dieting and trying to change our body to fit a mold that honestly is not diverse and was never created for us.

The data on the Latino population always lumps us all together, not taking into account that we aren't a monolithic group. Education, income, housing, and more all play roles in our health; therefore, telling someone that because they are Latino, they have a higher genetic risk of diabetes without accounting for the environmental triggers that can lead to a diagnosis is lazy and doesn't provide the full picture.

Medical Care, 11 Percent

After you've read the previous pages, I'm sure you know that access to healthcare also plays a big role in our health. Language barriers, immigration status, health literacy, and fear of being judged for one's weight all impact whether you will have access to medical care when you're sick or even for just yearly visits. If you work two or three jobs to make ends meet, or if your job cuts your hours so they do not have to give you medical insurance, or if your clinic doesn't have interpreters, or if you get judged for your size every time you walk into an office, your health will be affected. And consider your degree of health literacy—if you don't know how to read your labs, then you don't know what they mean and you cannot properly advocate for yourself.

You are less likely to get preventative care to help your health when you do not have access. But in our society, we blame the individual for not seeking care and not these real issues affecting our communities, so these diseases are perpetuated. We do not talk about not being able to take days off because you lack child-care or you're saving your PTO for the kids' appointments instead. We do not talk about the pressures many people face that have a tremendous impact on them.

For Gloria, her lack of dental insurance benefits and the time to attend appointments made dental care impossible, and her teeth suffered. This all directly affected her ability to carry out nutrition shifts.

Then of course there's when doctors shame you for eating fast food when that is all that's in your neighborhood, or they shame you for eating arroz blanco or tortillas, which are part of your culture. It's a vicious cycle of knowing you need healthcare but being afraid to be shamed. No one deserves this, and medical providers should treat everyone with dignity and respect.

I bring up weight stigma and shaming because I can hear many of you saying, *But I have access,* or, *I have insurance.* Weight stigma is the condition of being discriminated against or shamed because of one's weight. It is walking into a doctor's office and being told to lose weight when you're there because your elbow hurts. It is having perfect lab work and still being told you should lose a few pounds. It is the perception that only thin individuals can be healthy. It's associating laziness with fatness. It's families being denied in vitro fertilization (IVF) or adoption due to weight. It is *everywhere.*

It's the experiences of chulas like Sofia, who was in a horrible car accident and lost mobility in one leg and had four surgeries in three months, and when she *finally* walked on her own into her doctor's office, she was told she needed to lose weight and stop eating tortillas because her blood sugar was slightly elevated. The doctor took one look at her and saw her in a bigger body and immediately assumed her blood sugar being elevated was due to her weight. Not once did this doctor ask about her health, movement, or even the accident. The medications she was on? The stress? The trauma? The bed rest? *Nothing.* They just assumed that because Sofia is Mexicana, she should stop eating tortillas and move more.

But Sofia could not move more because she was still in pain. She was still recovering. She was mostly bedridden; she was *stressed.* And she barely ate tortillas, maybe once or twice a week, not daily. And when she did, they often were made by her mami from scratch. These assumptions not only hurt Sofia but also compromised the care she received. This story is not uncommon, and patients continue to suffer.

Physical Environment, 7 Percent

Now, as I mentioned above, 7 percent of the social determinants of health are attributed to access to food and housing and exposure to crime. In lower-income communities, access to fresh fruits and vegetables is poor. It is alarming that Latinos are two and a half times more likely to be food insecure, and 18.5 percent of Latino children experienced food insecurity in 2021.[5]

When we think about the communities into which Latinos immigrate in the United States, we can't overlook the importance of an absence of supermarkets and the fact that many live in what we are now calling food swamps under food apartheid. "Food apartheid" is defined by Karen Washington, cofounder of Black Urban Growers and co-owner of Rise and Root Farm, as "a system of segregation that divides those with access to an abundance of nutritious food and those who have been denied that access due to systemic injustice."[6]

These are the harsh and unfortunate conditions that many in the Latino community face. Yet, health statistics are often presented without context, failing to show how greater access to resources—such as healthcare, nutritious food, and safe living environments—can significantly lower the risk of disease. No, we all get lumped in together. We are told it is our fault and our foods, not the systems we live under, that are making us sick. So when I am educating our communities as a medical professional, my job is not to shame, but to help them find access to better foods. To help them go back to eating our delicious and nutritious foods and to *add* nutrition, not take anything away, because there already is a lack of it in our communities.

In Indigenous cultures, health has a lot to do with community. These cultures were the foundations of many of our families and upbringing. In the United States, health is extremely individualized and focused on pointing the finger at what you are doing wrong. But your health isn't determined by just food and movement decisions. As you saw with Gloria, there are countless factors impacting one's ability to experience good health.

If Gloria had been able to access more community resources without shame and guilt, if she was able to feel comfortable asking for help instead of feeling like a burden, her health would never have deteriorated to the point that it had when she walked into my office. Thankfully, my many connections at local nonprofits, the absence of a language barrier, and Gloria's sense of safety with me allowed me to get her to a dentist so her dental health could improve. As for nutrition, while we were waiting for the dental work, we focused on foods that she could make ahead of time, particularly with mangu being one of her favorites. We talked about mashing the egg into it so she could get that nutrition. We discussed making a broth of beans and rice. Being Dominican myself, I was able to suggest foods that we give to babies with no teeth that she could actually make herself. That thought had never crossed her mind.

This is why working with someone who isn't going to shame you is key. And if you are a medical provider reading this book, I truly hope you take the time to learn to be culturally humble, to talk to your patients as humans and to get to know them.

When it comes to honoring our bodies and health, I really want you to see that so much affects us. If it was as simple as "eat like this" and "move like that," life would be easy and we would all be healthy. But life is unpredictable, and we need to do what we can with what we have. To focus on the things we can work on and build small, healthy behaviors into our days to help reduce stress. Honoring our bodies and health is about realizing what is in our control and doing what is right for us.

Whether you are like Gloria or Sofia, finding helpful resources is essential. Navigating life with greater self-compassion and less guilt is key. You have the power to explore and take advantage of the community programs available to you. Seek out doctors and healthcare providers who will truly listen to your needs. Prioritize your health and well-being while also working to reduce stress.

TLDR: SDoH impact our entire existence and pursuit of health, and we need to have grace with ourselves.

CHULA PRACTICE: Practice understanding that we do what we can with what we have. We do not and cannot have control over everything. Focus on things that are in your control, such as:

1. Not skipping meals if possible
2. Staying hydrated
3. Trying to reduce stress
4. Focusing on sleep
5. Prioritizing walking more and sitting less

7

UNDERSTAND
YOUR NEEDS

Chula Story: Carmen

CARMEN ·is a first-gen Latina in her early thirties. When she was young, she became used to parenting herself and always did her best to meet people's expectations. As an adult, she came to realize that her self-worth, health, and even her ability to be a good mom were tied up in appearances. Carmen is the mom who makes amazing cakes and foods for her kids, but then she's on the side drinking a shake instead of enjoying the food and time *with* her kids. She was so worried about fulfilling the image of a good mom, but was she ever meeting her own mental, physical, or emotional needs? At what cost to herself was she trying to be the perfect mother?

I am a first-gen Dominican American who grew up as the eldest daughter of immigrant parents, which means I was translating all sorts of medical documents and mail since I learned how to read, which I guess made me mature for my age. Now I know it just means I was parentified. It also meant that none of us were meeting our needs and that there was *a lot* of scarcity mentality, forcing me into a caregiver role far too early.

In an article for HipLatina, Dr. Lisette Sanchez[1] says, "One of the challenges with parentification is that the children are also expected to hold the emotional stress that is tied to these experiences. The stress of translating a scary medical diagnosis or the fear of making a mistake on an important government form. At times also being burdened with the emotions of their parents."

Can we all just exhale and let that sink the fuck in. We were obliged to be little adults. A part of me mourns my lack of a childhood because I was always the third adult. However, I was never asked to parent my brothers, because my mom was a stay-at-home mom who was always there, so in many ways, we had a lot of privilege. My dad had a successful business he could run without needing to know much English, but the burden of translating medical, business, and legal documents was always on me. I even had to translate at parent-teacher conferences not only for myself but also for my younger brothers. I did have a little break in these responsibilities when we moved to Miami and most teachers and community leaders were bilingual, but once we came back to Philly, I was back to being an adult. You might be asking, *What the heck does any of this have to do with nutrition?* And the answer is *a lot.*

Because we always had to be aware of everyone else's needs, we probably were never aware of our own. I can guarantee that you heard at some point in your childhood, "Do as I say, not as I do," or "No preguntes, solo hazlo." We have always been told not to feel, not to talk back, not to even think of having preferences because children have zero say in our communities but are still expected to be adults when needed.

And listen, two truths can be true—our parents loved us very much and they fucked us royally when it comes to understanding our own needs. There are two ways to explain this. One is through understanding Maslow's hierarchy of needs.

MASLOW'S HIERARCHY OF NEEDS

Abraham Maslow, an American psychologist, created Maslow's hierarchy of needs to show the importance of having our most basic needs met in order to reach self-actualization. His hierarchy of needs provides a structured way to understand human motivation and well-being, outlining why it's crucial for certain needs to be met so that an individual can achieve their full potential.[*]

When I'm working with my chulas, I often use this to help them first heal their relationship with their needs so they can then heal their relationship with food. While the connection might not seem obvious on the surface, our ability to understand our needs plays into how healthy our relationship with food will be. This is specifically related to the conditioning that's been done in our communities, on both the systemic and interpersonal levels.

Let's take a look at what the hierarchy of needs is and the struggles that our community often faces in meeting them.

MASLOW'S HIERARCHY OF NEEDS VERSUS CHALLENGES IN THE LATINE COMMUNITY		
Maslow's Levels	General Description	Challenges in the Latinx Community
1. Basic Needs (Bottom Level)	Having food and water for sustenance and a safe place to live	• Food swamps: Living in areas where we have difficulty in accessing affordable, good-quality, fresh food

[*] Nuance Note: I think it's important to realize that although you may have what you need to become the most authentic version of yourself, genetics still play a role in our health. You can do *everything* "correctly" and still get sick. Be compassionate with yourself; we can only do so much.

MASLOW'S HIERARCHY OF NEEDS VERSUS CHALLENGES IN THE LATINE COMMUNITY		
Maslow's Levels	General Description	Challenges in the Latinx Community
		• Income status: Having a low income affects the fulfilling of basic needs • Housing: Gentrification, sub-par conditions • Language barrier: Communication issues with those who provide essential services
2. Feeling Safe and Secure	Feeling protected, not being in danger	• Immigration status: Fear of deportation causes stress and insecurity • Housing: High levels of crime and policing affect safety
3. Love and Belonging	Having friends and family for support; feeling like part of a community	• Discrimination and stereotyping: Social stigma affects the sense of belonging
4. Feeling Good About Yourself	Having healthy self-esteem and pride in accomplishments	• Systemic challenges: Systemic racism affects educational and job opportunities, impacting self-esteem • Familial expectations: First-gen children are expected to fulfill the American Dream
5. Reaching Your Full Potential	Achieving self-actualization; being the best you can be	• Income and immigration status: Limited income and uncertain immigration status inhibit focusing on personal growth

According to Maslow, we must satisfy the more basic needs at the bottom of the hierarchy before we can fully engage with the needs higher up. For instance, the pursuit of dreams and ambitions often takes a back seat when one is struggling with basic needs like food and safety.

In the Latine community, however, the journey up Maslow's pyramid comes with additional issues that complicate the ability to live a fulfilled life. At the most fundamental level of Basic Needs, there are several obstacles. Food deserts—areas with limited access to affordable, high-quality fresh food—are not uncommon in BIPOC communities. The issue of having a low income further exacerbates this, making it difficult for individuals to secure basic essentials like food, water, and safe housing. And on the topic of housing, issues like gentrification often displace families, forcing them to live in less-than-ideal conditions. Even basic communication is an issue due to language barriers, which makes accessing healthcare and education a challenge.

At the second level is Feeling Safe and Secure, which means feeling protected and not in danger. Unfortunately, undocumented immigrants within our community face the constant stress and insecurity that come with the fear of deportation. Plus, high crime rates and overpolicing in some areas make safety a day-to-day concern.

The third level, Love and Belonging, is often complicated by issues of discrimination and social stigmatization. While it is important to feel like we're part of a community and have support from friends and family, BIPOC communities, including Latine individuals, often must navigate a world where they face systemic bias. Constantly being met with the feeling of being "othered" can impact our sense of belonging and acceptance and exacerbate the negative repercussions of experiencing this. As a first-gen, I'm challenged by not feeling Dominican enough or American enough. Memories that come to mind are my primas always calling me the blanquita because I was the first of the cousins to be born in America and my English had no accent. On the other hand, I grew up with mostly white friends who would always refer to me as their "colored friend." It's as if I was never enough for either of these two parts of me, and I spent years wondering if I was ever going to feel that sense of belonging that I craved.

The fourth level, Feeling Good About Yourself, also known as self-esteem, introduces challenges related to systemic racism that affect educational and job opportunities. The lack of equitable opportunities impacts self-esteem and makes it hard to feel accomplished.

A notable example of this is the Doll Test, a study conducted by psychologists Kenneth and Mamie Clark that revealed the negative impacts of prejudice, discrimination, and segregation on African American children's self-esteem. It showed that a majority of the Black children tested, when given a choice between a Black or white doll, picked the white doll. In addition, they attributed positive traits to the white dolls over the Black dolls. This study was used in arguing *Brown vs. Board of Education,* which ruled school segregation unconstitutional, and it highlights the connection between lower self-esteem and systemic racism. In essence, being othered makes us feel inadequate at any age, affecting how we view ourselves and our self-worth. This also directly relates to imposter syndrome, which somehow always has a seat at the table even though we never invited it. More specifically, when your cultural foods and your body type are othered and made to seem different, it is understandable that you might lack confidence about your nutrition and body image.

Lastly, at the top of the pyramid is Reaching Your Full Potential, self-actualization. We all want to be the best that we can be, but it can be difficult to focus on our personal growth and obtaining long-term dreams when we have limited income or stress from having an uncertain immigration status.

Maslow's hierarchy serves as a general guide to human needs, but when societal and systemic challenges make it difficult for individuals to meet their needs at the lower levels of the pyramid, reaching the higher levels becomes increasingly difficult, especially for marginalized communities.

Addressing these systemic challenges is crucial for making it possible for everyone, regardless of their background, to satisfy their fundamental needs and reach their full potential. Another common challenge in immigrant communities is when your familia is trying to take care of not only themselves, but also the ones back home. A paycheck often doesn't go just to the person who earned that money; some of it also goes to the family back in their home country, who are counting on the worker to help them make ends meet. There's constant pressure to be the one everyone looks up to—financially and emotionally.

Moving up the pyramid was not available to us because our familia had to hustle and work hard and there was no time to focus on achieving our personal aspirations. Therefore, we struggle. We struggle with self-care and self-compassion. We struggle to move up. Some of us are definitely trying. We are going to therapy, we are healing our inner child, but shit, it is hard, and understanding our needs is *hard* because we are always taught to put others first, to take care of others first. Eating, exercising, and taking care of our health are privileges that many are not afforded.

MARIANISMO

Marianismo is a cultural concept within the Latine community and some other Catholic cultures. It is the opposite of machismo. In a review of Latin American politics, Nikhil Kumar, a copy editor at *Brown Political Review*,[2] explains that "machismo is a Latin American cultural analog to patriarchy: It refers to a set of hypermasculine characteristics and their value in traditional Latin American society." While machismo is all about being dominant and "manly," marianismo emphasizes the virtuous and pure roles that women are traditionally supposed to adopt. It's all about how close to the Virgen Maria we can be. In other words, we need to be pure, maternal, submissive, and self-sacrificing. Women are often seen as the caretakers and moral backbone of the family, the ones responsible for maintaining family unity and virtue. This is the very concept that we see at work in Carmen's experience.

As Latinas, we have the added pressure to be santa and pure, the perfect wife and mother, and always, above all, to put everyone in front of us, even if that means sacrificing ourselves. Essentially, when women fall into the role of marianista, all other genders by default have to assume a counter-role, reinforcing machismo. Marianismo and machismo rely on each other to maintain traditional power dynamics, where women are nurturing and self-sacrificing, and men are dominant. If both genders took on the same role, it would disrupt the expected structure that these cultural norms depend on. As a result, marianismo affects not just women but all genders, shaping how they function in society.

One of the first ways that a girl is exposed to this value is at quinceañeras. These celebrations were created as a way to present girls to society, signifying that they were ready to marry and were sexually mature enough to carry children. And I cannot even deal with the concept, honestly. I never want to shame anyone who had one, who wants to have one for their kid, or who really believes in this tradition, but I believe it's important that we know the origin of this tradition, although I do think the meaning is completely different now. We aren't able to grow, heal, or undo harm without knowing the real histories of our traditions.

But enough of my sidebar rant. Back to marianismo.

Characteristics Often Associated with Marianismo:

- **Submissiveness:** Women are encouraged to be submissive and deferential toward men in ways like serving food to the men in the family before the women, or giving men bigger plates. This reinforces traditional gender roles.
- **Virtue and purity:** Sexual purity and moral uprightness are highly valued. This often results in propagating misguided beliefs such as that you must be a virgin when you get married, or that using a tampon or riding a bike can take away your virginity, or that if you don't bleed after your first time, you were not a virgin because your hymen was already broken. I can go on and on about ways our sexuality is tied to purity.
- **Self-sacrifice:** Your kids and husband go first, always before your needs. You must give it all and leave nothing for yourself. Self-care is selfish.
- **Maternal role:** You are a mama first, a person last. The only purpose of your body is to reproduce. If you choose not to do so, you are being selfish.

These hetero norms are really complicated for LGBTQIA+ communities. Because of the heavy influence of Catholicism, not having a heteronormative identity directly conflicts with the patriarchy. If you aren't a cis, straight woman, according to marianismo, you can never accomplish what's expected of a woman. This is something that needs to be challenged more in our culture.

I want to bring all of this together because I know you are thinking, *Shit, Dalina, that was a lot and I need a fucking minute to absorb it all, but what does it have to do with nutrition and this book?* Well, these cultural norms teach us that our bodies are not ours—instead, they basically exist to serve the needs of men, and therefore we're always expected to sacrifice our needs.

Marianismo culture can lead to us wanting to be the "ideal" woman and make us believe that to be seen as perfect in our families' eyes—that is, as "wife material"—we need to conform to specific standards that include not just behavior but also appearance. This puts pressure on us to meet unrealistic body standards, which may contribute to body dissatisfaction or even eating disorders. When most women talk about their prime body, it's their teenage body, literally a child's body, that they're idolizing. This leads to us constantly wanting to shrink in order to fit into high-school jeans. But news flash: You were a child then, and now that you are a grown-ass adult, your hips are probably wider and that is okay.

The stress of trying to conform to such restrictive cultural standards of beauty and purity can be a significant factor in the development of eating disorders like anorexia, bulimia, and binge-eating disorder. Eating disorders are often kept secret, especially in a culture that emphasizes purity and control, where admitting to a "loss of control" over your eating habits can feel like a taboo, causing further emotional distress. To learn more about how purity culture and religious trauma can lead to eating disorders, Gloria Lucas over at Nalgona Positivity Pride is an amazing resource. I highly recommend reading her stuff and taking her webinars.

Now, I know that all of this was really hard to read, like really hard. For many of us, myself included, coming to terms with our parentification, navigating the challenges of moving up the ladder of needs, and coping with marianismo is a lot. I love my parents and am forever grateful for every single opportunity I have been afforded because they left their country and everything else behind so I could have a better life than them, and I do. But it doesn't mean that I am not struggling to self-actualize, or that marianismo and purity culture haven't fucked me up.

My kids are my *life,* and I know that the only way to take care of them is by taking care of myself because you cannot pour out of an empty cup. But the mom guilt is real. When I was a kid, my parents would sometimes yell at me and my siblings, and many times I didn't understand why they were yelling. It always felt harsh and angry when I wished they'd explain what I had done wrong. I knew that when I became a mom, I didn't want to confuse my kids by yelling at them and not explaining why. Now, as a mom, I try to meet my kids where they are, but sometimes I still yell. But instead of being hard on myself about not being perfect, I just let them know when I am wrong and apologize for my behavior. I've had to work very hard to unlearn the cultural norms that apply to me as a woman and as a mother. Wanting to be perfect is suffocating, and the constant pressure to conform to beauty standards that are meant to sell me to a man is *a lot*, but I'm working hard to undo those types of expectations.

Now that we have learned how we've been conditioned to put others before ourselves, we need to try to let go of those ideas and instead focus on our own needs.

UNDERSTANDING YOUR NEEDS

How do the chulas like Carmen start understanding their needs? The first step is recognizing the influence of the patriarchy on how you identify your needs. Often we are doing the best we can with the information that's been given to us and are practicing what our families have taught us. Without judging our upbringing, we need to question whether this type of thinking and these traditions are serving us. A great place to practice this is with food. Truly, we need to. There can be so much stress around food, especially when it's the last thing we have time for. Take a look at Carmen. She was so focused on being a great mom that she didn't have time to commit to herself. She didn't consider her own eating habits because she was preoccupied with feeding her kids. She felt that she had to meet her kids' needs first and then she could take care of herself, but by the time she got to herself, she had barely any energy left, so she would resign herself to having a shake. But since the shake was never enough to satisfy her, she would sneak sweets as well, a habit she hid from her children because she felt ashamed and didn't want them doing the same.

She recognized she didn't want to continue these behaviors and pass them on to her children. They deserved—and she deserved— to have a better relationship with food. But if she wanted to help her kids with that, she first needed to address her own needs and heal *her* relationship with it.

When I worked with Carmen, one of the first things she told me was that she was "addicted to food." It was how she explained her habit of constantly going for the sweets. At the heart of Carmen's addiction to sweets was her unmet needs. She was relying on the quick burst of tasty, enjoyable sweetness to experience something positive amid her stress. Food became her coping mechanism.

People commonly label themselves as "addicted to food" when they are actually using food to cope with stress and a lack of boundaries that have them feeling burned out. In many of these cases, what they need to do first is to look at their needs, identify their coping skills, and address their people-pleasing behaviors. People like Carmen should start with the ways they treat themselves as individuals. When you start to address your needs, it can be helpful to practice the strategy of "1 percent lifts." For example, for someone who is feeling stressed and burned out, 1 percent lifts can look like:

- Prioritizing a snack between meals instead of working through a stressful day without fuel

- Asking yourself what ingredient you can add to a meal to make it more satisfying
- Taking a break from a stressful workday or a busy moment to go outside and maybe take a short walk
- Filling up your water bottle and leaving it at your desk for when you are working

FOOD ADDICTION—WHAT IS REALLY AT PLAY?

No, you aren't addicted to ice cream or chips and salsa, but you are enamored with it. This happens particularly when you have never allowed yourself to have it regularly and without strings attached. Often when you have not eaten all day (likely because you have been meeting other people's needs) and that easily accessible food is finally in front of you, you find yourself eating quickly, with an almost out-of-control feeling. Maybe you have never cultivated a relationship with food or sugar in which it just is normal to have them. For your whole life it's been about being good, about burning off the calories and restricting. You have never been allowed to eat unconditionally, without rules. And chula, that is fucking scary. And I get it, it prob feels like you are letting yourself go.

This is exactly how Carmen felt when I asked her to start buying the foods she insisted she was addicted to. Her fear was that she would lose all control. While there are social media posts from thin, white Intuitive Eating dietitians that promise this tactic is the golden ticket to food freedom, I want to acknowledge that it is really scary to find yourself bingeing on Oreos. But remember this: As you begin to honor your needs by taking time for yourself and having balanced meals and snacks throughout the day, this kind of behavior can finally decrease.

Carmen's experience should remind you to avoid falling into

the trap of "fuck this," which is the feeling of all-or-nothing thinking—that is, either you eat all the cookies or you stop buying them entirely. I meet so many chulas who tell me that not controlling their food (what they called intuitive eating) didn't "work" and they let themselves go, which is just how Carmen felt.

Maybe you went from one extreme to another. You swung with the pendulum from one side (restrictive diets) to the other (*Fuck it, I'm gonna go buck wild*). And if you have not noticed it yet, extremes are not healthy or okay.

We want the pendulum to always be in the middle and never swinging to the extremes. Life happens in the middle. On some days you don't eat so many veggies. On others you are all veggied out. On some days you have a little more added sugar than usual, and on other days you might have none. You live life in balance, in the middle, not sweating it. Now you are probably wondering *How the fuck do I get there, Dalina? I need balance!* The answer is by creating habituation.

Food Habituation

Habituation with food is when repeated exposure to a particular food decreases one's physiological and emotional responses to it. Basically, the more access you have to it, the less control the food has over you. I heard Evelyn Tribole, the codeveloper of Intuitive Eating, speak about this on a podcast once. Think of habituation like you think of love or being enamored with someone. When you first meet that person, los corazones palpitan and your stomach is full of mariposas and all you want to do is be with this person. Once you drop that L-word, phew, is there anything better than hearing them say "Te amo"? It's literally like a drug. All you want to do is be with this person and say I love you a trillion times. But after a while, el amor is there but you don't have to say it twenty-seven times an hour. You can go days without saying it and you know you love them. That's habituation.

Here are a few ways you can start creating food habituation.

- **Allow yourself to have the foods.** This does not mean that you will eat five donuts in one sitting. You are probably going to feel sick. You will probably have a stomachache and feel like pure basura, and what is the point of that? You need to remind yourself that you as a grown-ass adult, one who is in her Señora era, can drink her cafecito and have a donut without guilt.
- **Remember that you can always come back for more.** When you begin the process of habituation and you have the foods around, remember that you can always come back for more. No, you do not need to eat the five donuts, but if after one donut you want another, you can have it. Or you can say, *Nah, I am okay.* But if in five minutes you do want another one, who's going to stop you? You are an adult, you can have it. You can always have them, but not to the point that will make you sick. Do you see the difference? And if you feel like you are truly out of control, please seek professional help, because this can be a sign of an eating disorder.
- **Add nutrition.** In Chapter 4, we talked about MyPlate and what a complete meal looks like. Who says a donut or pan dulce can't be part of your meal? A donut or pan dulce alone is just a lot of simple carbs that your body will run through very quickly. Instead, why not add protein and fruit? Have a full meal. If you do this, you will not feel so hungry that you want more donuts because you'll be satisfied and full. And if you choose to have the donut as a quick snack and you know

you are going to have a meal in an hour or two so you feel no need to add nutrition, that is okay too. Not every meal has to be complete; just know you will get hungrier quicker. But as a rule of thumb, always ask yourself, *Can I add nutrition to this?* And *you* get to decide if you want to.

Ultimately, Carmen needed to first address her needs. What she needed wasn't to stop buying the foods she was "addicted" to; what she needed was to recognize why she found herself going for those same foods time and again—because they were easy and convenient, and at the end of a long day of doing everything for her kids, she couldn't muster the energy to do more than that for herself.

TLDR: It's important to recognize that there are systems in place both outside of and within our culture that create barriers for our community to achieve our overall needs. We have been conditioned by marianismo culture to put everybody else before our own needs, but that needs to stop now. Recenter what you need and make time for yourself. Building habituation is key. Working with people who will help you find that is key. It is not a free-for-all. You certainly can eat, and eat what you love—allow yourself to do that. But if it's leading to bingeing and hurting your health, that is not making peace with food.

CHULA PRACTICE: Take five minutes for yourself today—do something that brings you joy! For example:

1. Walk around the block
2. Water your plants
3. Stand in the sun
4. Listen to your favorite song
5. Prep your favorite snack
6. Get a coloring book and color
7. Buy one food you really enjoy (even if you are afraid to have it in your house) and have it with a meal or as a snack

8

LISTEN TO YOUR
HUNGER AND FULLNESS

Chula Story: Valentina

VALENTINA is a professor with a self-described "neurospicy" brain who works a traditional academic job. Valentina was diagnosed with ADHD later in life, which she found both affirming of her symptoms and confusing for her identity. Valentina joined my Chula Club because she was dealing with low energy, stress, and a habit of going for hours without eating. She "couldn't feel hunger" and was overall struggling with making meals. In order to do her job, she was taking an ADHD medication that diminished her hunger cues, and she found that she often had waves of loving a specific meal (a hyperfixation meal, as the girlies say), only to hate it weeks later. I realized that she was having trouble learning how to listen to her hunger and fullness.

Hunger and fullness are both essential aspects of being human. Hunger literally means you are alive and your body needs energy, aka calories. It means your blood sugar has dropped and your body now needs energy (glucose) to get you through the day. But diet culture has taught us that being hungry is wrong. Diet culture sounds like, "Girl, you just ate air, how can you be hungry?" Both hunger and fullness send chills down some people's spines. And I am here to take that fear away.

For this, let's use the hunger scale.

Now, I am sure you have heard of the hunger scale, because people use it as a diet. They tell you, *Eat when you are hungry and stop when you are full.* Which is bullshit cuz 99 percent of y'all don't even know when you're hungry or full, and it can lead to the binge-and-restrict cycle. Instead, we will use this scale to guide you through some sensations and cues that will help you reconnect with your hunger and fullness.

Hunger or Fullness Level	What It Means	Real Life	Nuance
Level 1— Painfully Hungry	Your blood sugar has dipped so low that to get your attention your body is sending you pain signals, usually in the form of a headache or even stomach pains.	You should not feel pain when hungry, but we have been conditioned to think that eating less is more and that hunger is bad, and so we have become disconnected from our cues. Sometimes pain is the only way the body knows to send a signal.	Take a deep breath, stop, and go eat something.

Hunger or Fullness Level	What It Means	Real Life	Nuance
Level 2— Hangry	You have hypoglycemia, a clinical term meaning your blood sugar has dipped really low—it's probably about 70—and your body is HANGRY. Your body needs energy ASAP.	Well, you are certainly not yourself when you are hangry! That Snickers commercial did not lie, but this hunger is not normal. It is primal. Your body needs energy quickly, and that energy is sugar. And you will not crave a kale smoothie, you will want something that will give you energy quickly. You will reach for the sugariest food you can find. And you will eat it. You will eat it until you are overly full.	Now, this is where many of you think hunger starts, but it is not. Hunger starts before this. This is when you have waited too long to satisfy it. You do not want to get here. You should be eating every three to four hours to make sure your body has energy!

Hunger or Fullness Level	What It Means	Real Life	Nuance
Level 3—Hungry	Your body is communicating with you via hunger cues that it is time to eat.	This is the classic feeling of hunger: a rumble in your stomach, feeling ready to eat, and noticing your energy levels dropping. Your stomach starts growling, you might feel tired. This, however, despite what diet culture tells you, is not thirst. You do not confuse pee and poop, so you should not confuse hunger and thirst! The line between levels 2 and 3 can be crossed quickly.	This is where many of you will drink water, because diet culture has told you you're not hungry, you are thirsty. So you drink water, which creates a sense of fullness as your stomach expands and makes space for the water. However, it is not a true and lasting sense of fullness. You are essentially tricking your body into not sending you hunger signals so you will not eat. But 15 to 30 minutes later, when your stomach has emptied, your body is like, *Wtf?* And now you are HANGRY, and you know what happens then.

Hunger or Fullness Level	What It Means	Real Life	Nuance
Level 4— Feeling Like You Can Eat	These are the actual first signs of hunger.	It's when you should start preparing to eat. You might notice that you cannot get that last sentence in the email right because you cannot concentrate. Or that food thoughts are running through your head. Or that smells are heightened. Or that you're salivating. Basically, you are tired; your energy is dipping.	Now, this is where I know you grab the cafecito because you can't concentrate, effectively shutting down the hunger cues. But, chula, this is not when to do that. Because that will make you hangry, and you know how that goes. Take a break, wrap up the email. Order lunch or start warming it up. Get ready to eat. You will be more productive if you eat.
Level 5— Chilling, Not Hungry or Full	There are no signs of hunger or fullness; you're just chilling.	This is when you don't feel any need for food because you either just ate a few hours ago and have zero sensations in the belly or you started eating and your hunger has stopped but you are not full.	This is between meals. This is where practical hunger would kick in if needed. I will talk more about practical hunger later in this chapter.

Hunger or Fullness Level	What It Means	Real Life	Nuance
Level 6— Stomach Feels Full, but Not Satisfied	You are full, but not satisfied.	This is while you are eating. You start to feel full, but you are not done eating; you might still be only a few bites in. But you're not fully full, and you are definitely not satisfied.	Most diets tell you to stop here. And this is probably why you never feel full because you truly aren't full. You are stopping the eating process before you get all the calories–aka energy–you need. You are not satisfied, and this can backfire. This might also be when you stop because you ate something that wasn't bomb, meaning you ate it because you had it around, but it didn't satisfy you. And that is okay; not all food is going to be amazing. You will have meals that are blah, that leave you full but not satisfied. But you might find yourself wanting that satisfaction later.
Level 7— Stomach Feels Comfortable and Satisfied	You are full and satisfied.	You are full and satisfied. Mission complete.	No notes, you are good. The food was great, and you are comfortable. You feel good. Life is good. This is where we will usually stop eating.

Hunger or Fullness Level	What It Means	Real Life	Nuance
Level 8—Just a Little Too Full	You are a little over fullness.	You ate a little past fullness because you had the dessert or last few bites.	This is when you eat a little past fullness because you only had two bites left and that shit was so good you just wanted to finish it. You are past full, but you are not uncomfortable. This is sharing a dessert with friends or going for ice cream after a meal on a date. Are you wrong for eating past fullness? No. Will this happen often? Yes. Living life means that you will have these beautiful moments with food, and that's okay.
Level 9—Unbutton-Your-Pants Kinda Feeling	You are Thanksgiving full.	You ate too much and need to unbutton your pants.	We all know this feeling. You are uncomfortable because you overate. Are you bad because of it? No, but if you frequently start to eat at the hangry level, you will be here a lot and you will think this is a normal degree of fullness. It is not.

Hunger or Fullness Level	What It Means	Real Life	Nuance
Level 10— Extremely Uncomfortable	You are painfully full.	You have a stomachache or maybe diarrhea.	You don't want this. Eating should never be painful. This is an extreme end of the spectrum. Will it happen? Maybe. Should you feel guilt and shame if it does? No. Work on figuring out why you reached this fullness level and find some help. You don't have to do this alone.

Now, you will notice that hunger and fullness ebb and flow. It is not an exact science. You will not use this as a diet and then message me, *Omg I am so good, I always eat when I am hungry and stop when I am full.* That is neither realistic nor practical, especially if you're like Valentina.

There will be days when you are hangry. There will be days when you will eat past fullness. There will be days when you're not hungry at all. You will have days when breakfast was blah, lunch was bomb, and dinner was fine. You will learn to just live, not check off the numbers on the hunger scale. And you will learn to connect with your hunger and fullness cues so you can enjoy food.

Now, hunger is not always that simple. We are humans, after all, and sometimes you will have to eat even if you aren't hungry, or if you are having a rough fucking day and that ice cream will make you feel better. Or maybe you are at a party and your favorite tía made your fave dessert, so you decide to have some. All of this is normal. Taking pleasure in food is one of the things that make us human.

There are different types of hunger that I think we sometimes confuse for each other and don't really know what we want in that particular moment. If we're able to identify what type of hunger we're experiencing, we're better able to address the issue.

The types of hunger include:

- **Physical hunger:** You know that feeling when your stomach starts growling? That's your body telling you, "Hey, I need some fuel!" Physical hunger is like that primo who shows up on time, no drama. It gives you a heads-up with a stomach growl or even a little mood swing. Don't ignore this; feed it some love and some nutrients. You don't want to get to the "hangry" stage, do you?
- **Emotional hunger:** Emotional hunger is that tricky amiga who makes you feel like you gotta have that chocolate cake, like, right now. But, chula, emotional hunger is a diva, it wants what it wants, and usually it wants it ya mismo. It's all about those feelings, you know? Maybe you're stressed, maybe you're sad, or hey, maybe you're even happy. This is where you gotta pause. We don't want you numbing those hard emotions with food. Now, I'm not saying not to eat the cake. But you should know what's driving you *toward* eating the cake. Are you hoping to numb the feelings, or are you actually going to use the food to cope? Addressing or avoiding emotions with food is completely normal, and I'll get into it a bit more in the next chapter.
- **Social hunger:** Social hunger is that charismatic tía who convinces you to have just one more tamale, even if you're already full. You're at a party or a family get-together and everyone's eating, so you feel like you should be too. But it's

okay to say "No, gracias" if you do not want it. Eating in a social setting is a beautiful thing, but let it be on your terms. Enjoy the company, the chisme, and the comida, but listen to your body, not just the crowd. You are allowed to say yes, and you are allowed to say no. Do what is best for you.

- **Practical hunger:** This is like your abuela telling you to wear a sweater because it's going to be cold later. It's you eating now because you know you won't have a chance to later. You're not super hungry now, but you're being smart and planning ahead. If you struggle with a situation like Valentina's, honoring practical hunger is being proactive. Having a protein bar or a snack in your bag for if you get hungry is just like carrying a sweater in case you get cold. So go ahead, make that sandwich before your long meeting or eat a little something before running those errands. Trust me, your future self will thank you for it.

Fullness is complex, and as I explained above, it will ebb and flow. There is no right or wrong way to feel hunger or fullness, but many chulas I see do not know how to be comfortably full or can't tell what type of fullness they're experiencing.

The types of fullness:

- **Physical fullness:** Like I said above, this is when you feel that physical expansion in the belly.
- **Emotional fullness:** When we eat emotionally as a tool, we feel "full" when we feel better. More on this in the next chapter.
- **Social fullness:** This is when you use social cues to stop eating. Maybe you're at dinner with friends and although everyone else at the table has finished their food, you still have a bunch on your plate, but you can feel their eyes upon you to hurry up

so you all can go hit the bar afterwards. Feeling the pressure, you decide to stop even though physically you're not full. This is something that unfortunately often happens, and it can backfire if you are undereating.

Many things can interfere with our fullness and mess with our cues. Ask yourself whether you're eating enough in total. Or are you dieting on the DL? Some people try to fill up on Fiber One bars and diet and low-calorie foods. When you are eating so much fiber, it expands in your belly and you have the physical sensation of fullness, but you are not getting enough calories. This will cause you to feel hungry quicker and maybe even to binge.

Are you constantly following social fullness when you are out with friends, undereating and getting bland-ass salads because they are all on diets, and then getting home and eating a sleeve of Oreos? All of this affects our hunger and fullness cues. Many of us have ghosted them for so long that they've stopped trying to reach us.*

HORMONAL REGULATION OF HUNGER AND FULLNESS

As mentioned in Chapter 5, the endocrine system plays a critical role in regulating both hunger and fullness through the interplay of various hormones and neural signals.

I share these details with you because you always see influencers saying that your hormones are the reason for your health and

---

* This is an analogy that a fellow chula shared with me, and I think it's so spot-on in illustrating the importance of listening to our cues. If you've ghosted someone, you don't expect them to come back. It's important to be a good friend to your body's cues.

weight struggles. I want you to be educated and not fearful. An important caveat: If you have a condition that affects a specific hormone, you need to follow your doctor's recommendations for your illness. Nutrition fixes cannot make your body produce a hormone once it has stopped (for example, if your body needs insulin replacement, thyroid hormone medication may be an appropriate and needed treatment because the thyroid affects metabolism).

These hormones work together to help us, but they work properly only if we are eating enough; they can get jacked up when we are undernourishing ourselves and restricting our food intake. Your body is smart, and its goal is to survive, so instead of fearing hunger and fullness, we need to learn to connect with and listen to our body and its needs.

- **Ghrelin:** The "hunger hormone"; signals to the brain that it's time to eat
- **Insulin:** Regulates blood sugar and signals satiety, or fullness
- **Leptin:** Produced by fat cells; counters ghrelin's effects by signaling fullness
- **GLP-1 (glucagon-like peptide-1):** Stimulates insulin secretion and inhibits glucagon secretion, limiting changes in blood sugar before and after a meal
- **PYY (peptide YY):** Released after eating; reduces appetite
- **Cholecystokinin (CCK):** Produced by the intestines; helps to signal fullness and slows down gastric emptying
- **Cortisol:** The "stress hormone"; influences both hunger and fullness by promoting emotional eating and cravings for high-calorie foods

Honestly, listening to our bodies can be really hard when those of us in Latine households are trying to set boundaries around our hunger and fullness and there are so many family members who like to get all up in our business about what we're eating. Valentina struggled with this after she started working on eating smaller, more frequent meals to support her ADHD brain. One time, when she was visiting family, Valentina planned to have a balanced snack around five P.M., knowing her family had scheduled an eight P.M. dinner. When her mother saw her eating, she asked, "What are you doing? We have dinner at eight P.M." This was frustrating to Valentina because she was working to manage her hunger and fullness. Valentina learned from working with both her therapist and me that she could empower herself in these moments to set boundaries with her family.

I think a great way to start setting effective boundaries is by seeing a therapist. There are so many great therapists out there talking about how to do that.°

I don't know about you, but "setting boundaries" is a phrase en espanol that does not make sense to me. "Poner limites" does not translate correctly to me, pero I guess we have to aprender a poner estos limites anyway.

Next time you're at a family gathering and are offered food that you don't want, I urge you to communicate your boundaries to your familia. There's a way to do it that is both compassionate and firm. Here are some phrases you can use:

Thank you so much for offering me this flan, I am actually really full and if I eat it, I will be uncomfortable. Let me hold off a little bit before I eat it, or I will take it home. I don't want to feel uncomfortable and want to enjoy my time here.

Muchas gracias por ofrecerme este flan, la verdad es que ya estoy muy lleno/a y si lo como me voy a sentir incómodo/a.

° Two of my favorite therapists to learn from are Maria G. Sosa (@holistically grace) and Dr. Mariel Buqué (@dr.marielbuque).

Déjame esperar un poco antes de comerlo o me lo llevo a casa.
No quiero sentirme mal y quiero disfrutar mi tiempo aquí.

WOW, thanks for making me my favorite meal. I am actually
super full from eating earlier and I really want to enjoy it, you
know this dish is my favorite. Let me eat it when I am hungry.

¡WOW, gracias por prepararme mi plato favorito! La verdad
es que estoy bastante lleno/a porque comí hace poco y real-
mente quiero disfrutarlo, ya sabes que este plato me encanta.
Déjame comerlo cuando tenga hambre.

When you use "I" statements, you let them know how you feel and that it's not about them or their amazing meal, but that you do not want to be uncomfortable. Food is our love language in our culture, but we also never want to be malcriada; a no will often not be enough, because our communities are not used to us saying no as a full sentence. Explain how you feel and remember that boundaries are for you to set with others. They choose whether they want to uphold them, but that is not your problem. You should enforce them and move on.

I know that all of this is a lot to take in, and I want you to come back to this chapter as often as you need to. Setting boundaries with our familia can be difficult, but it's all in the name of listening to our bodies and achieving authentic health.

I want you to remember that eating is self-care. It's the ultimate act of self-care. It is you telling your body that it is safe, that you are taking care of it, and that you are listening. Valentina had to learn that, and she is still learning it. Even though Valentina takes medication that affects her appetite, she values her energy needs and the journey she has had to take to meet them. This is work that we all need to practice every day.

TLDR: Eating when you're hungry and nourishing yourself to fullness can be complicated, but it's necessary because it is about meeting your needs. Your hormones are not broken; they need energy to function. A key way to honor your hunger and fullness is by setting boundaries with those around you and yourself.

CHULA PRACTICE:

1. Practice connecting with hunger by allowing your body to feel other sensations.
   a. Walk on the grass with no shoes on. Feel the grass and the connection to the ground.
   b. Lie down for five minutes with a timer set and connect with the sensations as you tap your face, your belly, and your shoulders.
2. Try eating with connection. You don't have to be completely undistracted, but eat with the intention of connecting to what your body needs.
3. Practice "I" statements. Write them in your phone notes app or text them to someone you trust. You are not being malcriada by setting boundaries. Creating them should make you feel better.

Food Is Amor, and Yes, You Can Cope with It.

9

ACKNOWLEDGE
YOUR EMOTIONS

Chula Story: Emily

EMILY is a thirty-five-year-old realtor chula. She joined my group because she always found herself bingeing. She felt out of control around food and labeled herself "addicted to food and a stress eater." She wanted to fix this and stop her emotional eating. So I began to ask questions.

Emily grew up as a first-gen Puerto Rican American. Her parents worked multiple jobs, and as an only child, she was left alone a lot to fend for herself. Her parents would leave her money for dinner and tell her to order food and split it in half so she would have something to take to school the next day. And so, Emily grew up splitting everything she ate in half. As an adult, she found herself splitting every meal—no matter how hungry she was—in half. She developed a habit of "grazing" or eating sporadically throughout the day. She worked in real estate and was often showing houses or meeting deadlines, so her eating was not very consistent. But when she got home, she would pour herself a glass of wine and begin to cook (she loved cooking and found it therapeutic), and as she cooked, she would find herself snacking, drinking, and eating. She would finally sit down in front of her TV to relax and eat her whole meal, and then she would crave dessert. She felt so out of control, like she was bingeing. She joined my membership as a self-proclaimed binge eater, stress eater, and emotional eater.

If this sounds like you in any way, I want you to know that you are not alone. We throw the words "binge eater," "stress eater," and "emotional eater" around a lot, and we need to talk about them. Binge eating disorder (BED) is a serious eating disorder. If you sometimes eat a lot in one sitting, it does not mean you have BED, and I think it is super important to understand that. The American Psychiatric Association (APA) defines binge eating disorder as recurrent episodes of eating "abnormally large quantities" of food in a short period of time, with episodes marked by feelings of a lack of self-control, guilt, embarrassment, or disgust. People may binge eat alone to hide their behavior. To meet the APA criteria for a binge eating disorder diagnosis, the behavior must be associated with marked distress and occur an average of at least once a week over three months.

There is a difference between a serious condition like BED and you eating past fullness a few times a week. It is possible that you, chula, are just hangry. You are hangry because you have not eaten enough all day. You crave sugar because you have not eaten enough carbs over the day. You stress eat or emotionally eat because you ghosted your hunger all day and then you came home and relaxed and the hunger was finally able to surface.

Now, remember when we talked about the hunger scale and said that if you begin eating when you are hangry, you are going to be so hungry that you will most likely eat to an uncomfortable fullness? Well, when we are numbing our emotions with food, we do the same thing.

FOOD IS COMFORT, FOOD IS PLEASURE

Emotional eating is normal, and we all do it. However, it is often riddled with shame and guilt. It's considered the act of consuming food in response to a range of emotional states rather than out of physical hunger. Whether it's stress, sadness, loneliness, or even joy, people across cultures and of all ages frequently turn to food to feel better, but what I often see is that they end up numbing their feelings with it. This might happen because they didn't learn to acknowledge their emotions, so instead they eat them away and act like the feelings are not happening.

Let's revisit Emily's story. She grew up not only undereating because she split everything in half (which led to her always being starved by dinnertime!), but also never allowing herself to feel emotions. Growing up while mostly parenting herself and basically pulling herself up by the bootstraps (which is not fair for a child—or any adult, for that matter—to have to do alone), she was basically taught to just push through and not feel any emotions. She had to be strong, and she had to just do it. I invite you to read Prisca Dorcas Mojica Rodríguez's *For Brown Girls with Sharp Edges and Tender Hearts: A Love Letter to Women of Color* if you have not already. This is an amazing book if you want to understand how we as Latinas, as part of a Latino-Latine-Latinx community, have been sold an American Dream based on the myth of meritocracy. This is something that can be very hard for us to come to terms with, but when we realize it, we can see how it affects us not just with our work and having a hustle mentality, but also with food.

We fight our emotions all the time. We are told to conceal and not to feel. And in the process, we shut down our hunger cues and work through them. We are not allowed to feel our feelings. And when shit hits the ceiling, all we know how to do is eat to comfort ourselves. We are taught not to feel our feelings in any other way except than by numbing ourselves with food. And we do this because food is memories. Food is happiness, food is love. Coping by using food is natural; numbing with it is complicated.

However, this natural tendency to cope with food is often seen in a negative light. It's common to hear emotional eating described as "a lack of willpower," "emotional weakness," or even "a fast track to gaining weight." These labels can create a sense of shame or guilt, further complicating an individual's relationship with food and emotions.

The media plays a huge role in perpetuating these negative stereotypes. Dominated by diet culture and wellness trends, media narratives often categorize emotional eating as a "bad habit" in need of "fixing" or "control," thereby intensifying the stigma associated with it.

Think of any rom-com or kids' show you have ever watched. Every one of them has a pivotal scene where the main character has a horrible day or goes through an intense breakup, and what does this person do? They walk up to the freezer, grab four tubs of ice cream, and scream and cry. Chips and candy get smeared all over their face. They feel like a failure, they feel like they did something immoral, and now they are using food to numb it in not the healthiest way. I say "not the healthiest" because this person isn't trying to solve the issue, they are just numbing it by eating. After this pivotal scene, usually some sort of confidant tells them they need to snap out of it and focus on themselves. It then cuts to the person solving the problem by working out, eating healthy, and "fixing" their life. We have taught a generation of people that when they have a bad day they should binge, and when they finally fix themselves, they will be super healthy. There is no nuance in this representation of food used as a coping mechanism. Consuming food is a common coping mechanism; it's not about completely cutting it out of our life in that way. It's about learning to not take it to the extreme.

The role of food as a form of emotional and social support has been a cornerstone of human civilization for centuries. Sharing a meal has always been about more than just eating; it's a ritual that fosters community, nurtures relationships, and bolsters coping skills. Ancient cultures relied on communal feasts not only to celebrate victories but also to strengthen community spirits during challenging times. Similarly, the act of breaking bread together has been a sign of peace, alliance, and emotional connectedness in many societies.

Food also takes center stage in most of our lives' significant emotional events. There is literally not one culture that does not celebrate or mourn with food. From weddings to funerals, we have dishes for each occasion that bring joy or soothe our souls by telling stories and helping us remember. From my own culture, what specifically comes to mind is habichuela con dulce, which we eat only during semana santa (Easter week). In Mexico, the traditional celebration known as Dia de los Muertos honors the deceased. Some families travel to cemeteries to bring the deceased's favorite foods while others build altars to the dead in their homes. Among the main foods that are prepared and enjoyed are pan de muertos, tamales, pozole, sugar skulls, atole, and champurrado.

There are also festivals marking seasons or harvests that emphasize the emotional relationship humans have with food. During these festivals, food becomes more than just a product of a community's labor; it represents its collective hope, and often a shared sense of relief and gratitude for nature's bounty. Understanding the historical and cultural contexts in which emotional eating is embedded can help us appreciate it as a universal human experience. And we should learn how to use it as a tool to help us, not as a way of numbing ourselves.

It's crucial to acknowledge that emotional eating also has a biological basis, something that's often ignored when discussing its negative connotations. When we eat foods that we enjoy, particularly those that are rich in carbohydrates or fats, the brain releases neurotransmitters like serotonin that act as natural mood lifters. Remember when I said food is memory? This is what I meant: Food is associated with happy moments and its consumption releases serotonin, which is often called the "feel good" hormone and which plays a significant role in regulating our moods, emotions, and sleep. So when you are having a rough day and you crave your abuela's sancocho or ice cream, it makes perfect sense. Eating to cope with emotions doesn't indicate a lack of willpower; it's a biological response designed to make you feel better. And no, you are not addicted to it. You are simply human.

The Clean Your Plate Club

The "clean your plate" mantra is not unique to any one culture, but in the Latino community, it takes on specific nuances colored by tradition, family dynamics, and notions of respect and gratitude. Food is a central element in Latino culture, symbolic of love, family, and community. Meals are not just about nourishment, they are social events during which family bonds are strengthened. In this context, the act of cleaning your plate is less about the food and more about honoring the hands that prepared it. Leaving food on your plate might be interpreted as rejecting the love and effort put into making the meal and, by extension, as a slight to the family.

Additionally, many Latino families have roots in countries where food scarcity is or has been a concern, where wasting food is seen not only as disrespectful but also as a sign of privilege and ignorance about the value of resources. This background amplifies the significance of finishing the food on one's plate, transforming it into an act that transcends the immediate family and reflects broader issues of sustainability and respect for labor. The "clean your plate" mentality has complex layers of history, socioeconomic factors, and deep-rooted cultural values.

However, this mentality can also lead to challenges around emotional eating and body image, given that refusing food might cause familial tension or be seen as disrespectful. In a culture in which food is equated with love and social belonging, the emotional weight given to eating behaviors is particularly heavy. This can create a complex relationship with food that intersects with emotional well-being in intricate ways.

Understanding the cultural importance of cleaning your plate in the Latino community offers a more nuanced view of emotional eating. While the practice has its roots in meaningful traditions and values, its impact on individual choices about food and emotional health can be complex. Acknowledging these cultural factors can help in developing a more compassionate and nuanced approach to discussions around emotional eating, diet, and health within this community.

Survival

From an evolutionary perspective, emotional eating can be viewed as an adaptive survival mechanism too. Early human individuals who were better at storing energy in the form of fat were more likely to survive in harsh conditions where food was scarce. The stress response that drove our ancestors to consume more calories in preparation for fight-or-flight situations remains with us. This explains why when we were all stuck at home during COVID, so many of us got into the habit of baking and even hoarding food. Not because something was wrong, but because, from a fight-or-flight perspective, our stressed-out bodies thought we needed to consume extra calories to prepare us to either fight or flee. If you gained weight, you did not fail. Your body was protecting you and making sure you survived.

Emotional eating can also be viewed as a form of self-care. In a hectic, crazy fucking world, taking the time to sit down with a meal or snack that brings you joy can be a radical act of self-kindness and a way to feel safe, as I said in the previous chapter. If going through a global pandemic taught us anything, it's that things can literally change at the drop of a hat, and we should always have compassion for and take care of ourselves. The key is not numbing—instead, be fully present in the experience of eating and savoring every bite while working through whatever issue it is that's causing you distress. Allow yourself to feel the emotions and let the food soothe you. It can transform a simple meal into a deeply comforting ritual as you learn how to deal with the situation.

It's important to remember that while emotional eating is great, it's not a one-size-fits-all remedy. The objective is not to replace one form of emotional management with another, but to expand the tool kit. Emotional eating can coexist with other coping mechanisms like physical exercise, deep-breathing exercises, or talking through your emotions with friends or counselors. It's knowing that you can have a shitty day and want ice cream, but it doesn't have to be the whole tub. It can be a few scoops and a walk with a friend to talk things out. It's asking yourself, *What will make me feel better right now?* And that can be a combination of things. The goal isn't to forget the issue, but to work through it.

The Importance of Taking Satisfaction in Food

The importance of feeling satisfied with the food we eat is often overlooked in discussions about diet and emotional well-being, yet it serves a pivotal role. Satisfaction isn't merely about feeling full; it encompasses a holistic sense of pleasure, both physical and emotional. From the flavors that dance on your palate to the comforting warmth that spreads through you with a home-cooked meal, satisfaction goes beyond nourishment to tap into deeper psychological and even spiritual needs. Intriguingly, research[1] indicates that when we eat food that genuinely satisfies us, we actually digest it better. The digestive system is closely linked with the pleasure centers in the brain, optimizing nutrient absorption when we are contented and relaxed.[2] A study published in *Flavour* supports this by showing how pleasure activates brain mechanisms that regulate digestive processes, reinforcing the connection between satisfaction and better digestion.[3]

This idea dovetails beautifully with the concept of emotional eating and challenges the stigma surrounding it. I will repeat this because it's so important: Eating for emotional reasons can be a form of self-care, and when done mindfully, it adds to our sense of satisfaction and overall well-being. In a society that often weaponizes food—paradoxically promoting indulgent holiday feasts while chastising people for emotional eating—embracing satisfaction can be an act of personal empowerment.

This is especially true in culturally diverse settings like the Latine community, where food is not just fuel but a tapestry of family, tradition, and identity. Cleaning your plate in this context might be less about conforming to societal pressures and more about participating in a communal expression of love and respect. For some, preparing food is their love language and they may feel disrespected when you don't clean your plate. You can use "I" statements to support your boundaries while also holding empathy for the way your relative may feel.

Food has deeper meaning and value in many of our Latine

cultures that can fall by the wayside in the fast-paced, work-focused, profit-driven existence that we have in the United States. I think that's why finding satisfaction in food is both so important and so different in our cultures compared to the prevailing U.S. attitude.

I think so much of this goes back to meeting your needs. When you prepare satisfying food, you are telling yourself that you matter and your needs are worth meeting. As Latines, we value the foods we put on our tables because they're coming from a place of true nourishment: They take care of the body and they taste good.

It seems hard to do this as part of the mainstream culture of the United States, which emphasizes urgency and values doing tasks quickly.° But we can have both the convenience and the satisfaction by adding nutrition (fresh salsa, cremas, Tajín, etc.) to enhance the experience of eating convenience foods that are easy to prepare in the midst of our busy lives.

When we're talking about emotional eating, in a way, we are talking about slowing down enough to connect with ourselves. This is hard to do when you're settling down in a new country, working multiple jobs, raising your kids, and trying to maintain a healthy lifestyle.

We can embrace the slowness in our satisfying cultural dishes. In the DR, food was always affordable even for the poor. I can envision the men playing dominoes at the colmado, the ladies gossiping, and the children playing in the streets. Although things are different now, the work-life balance there hasn't changed in the way it has in the United States. My parents tell me that their friends back home aren't sick, that they're living their lives, as op-

---

° One place where we see this is in school lunchrooms, where the average time a child takes to eat is seven to ten minutes because we value work and grades over nourishment and play.

posed to the people I see in the United States. Yes, this is anecdotal evidence, but I think the takeaway message is that life is more satisfying there.

Chula, I'm not telling you to move out of the country. What I'm telling you to do is add flavor, to value sazón. Know that even in a moment when you're rushing, you can still slow down and add freshness, texture, spice, and nutrition. This creates satisfaction for us. We can make the best of what we have with inspiration from our cultures.

Reframing Emotional Eating

It's true that some of our most satisfying and flavorful foods are sources of joy as well as tools for emotional coping. Emotional eating is often framed as a negative behavior, but it's essential to remember that it can also be a valid form of self-care when approached mindfully. The key things to work on are balance and moderation. If you find that you consistently turn to food as your sole coping mechanism, it might be beneficial to diversify the ways you manage stress and emotional upheaval. This doesn't mean you have to give up the comfort that food can provide; instead, think of it as expanding your emotional tool kit. For instance, you might discover that physical exercise—be it a brisk walk, a jog, or a yoga session—can offer a different but equally effective form of relief. The endorphins released during physical activity can boost your mood and provide a sense of well-being.

Building a strong social support network is another healthy alternative. Sometimes the act of sharing your worries or joys with another human being can be incredibly cathartic. In moments when you're tempted to reach for comfort food, consider reaching out to a friend or family member for a quick chat. Of course, this isn't to say that you can't enjoy a piece of chocolate or your favorite snack while you talk! The point is to avoid relying solely on food to manage your emotional state. For those who find that their emotional struggles are severely impacting their quality of life, seeking professional help from a psychologist or counselor can provide specialized coping strategies and a confidential space to explore deeper emotional issues.

Another tip for healthy emotional eating is to opt for foods that not only satisfy your emotional cravings but also provide nutritional value. I am not telling you to make swaps or healthify your desserts or snacks. What I am suggesting is recognizing that eating to soothe your emotions does not mean the opposite of eating for nutrition. Choosing a piece of fruit, a bowl of yogurt, or a handful of nuts can offer both comfort and nourishment. That way, you're attending to your emotional needs while also taking care of your body. It's not about denying what you really want; it's about making choices that serve you on multiple levels. This isn't the only tip on emotional eating or the only way to emotionally eat. But it may serve you in certain situations.

There will be times—and it takes a while to understand this— when you'll see that food does not have to have a nutritional purpose every time we eat it. Sometimes, you will just want the tasty treat while you sit and relax on the couch after a long day of work. There is goodness in this, and this pause to meet your needs on a busy day is the way we start to heal.

By recognizing that emotional eating is a part of the human experience and expanding your repertoire of coping mechanisms, you can cultivate a more balanced, guilt-free relationship with food. Integrate exercise, social support, and even professional assistance into your emotional management strategies, and you'll find that emotional eating can exist as one of many options in a holistic approach to well-being.

Looking back at Emily's experience, we see that her emotional eating started to improve when she prioritized stopping for meals and really focusing on practical hunger during her busy schedule. She learned not to numb herself with food, but rather to use it as a tool of self-care instead. This meant that sometimes she did "eat" her feelings, but she also built a habit of preparing food for herself, slowing down around meals, and adding satisfaction to foods that she could prepare with ease after a busy day at work. It's about finding that balance.

TLDR: Emotional eating can be a self-care tool, but first we must learn not to numb ourselves with it. Living in the "both/and" means accepting that life will always bring stress, but we can choose how we cope. Emotional eating can coexist with other strategies, like mindful breathing, physical activity, or connecting with loved ones. By acknowledging our emotions rather than avoiding them, we can use emotional eating as one part of a broader, balanced approach to meeting our needs.

CHULA PRACTICE: You need to have multiple coping mechanisms—it can't just be food. Make a list of things that help you feel better.

- What can you do for playful fun? Coloring, dancing, singing?
- Intellectual fun? Puzzles, reading?
- Comfort? A weighted blanket, a comedy show, a hot bath or shower?
- Movement? Exercise?

Keep this list with you, in your phone notes, on your laptop, on a sticky note, anywhere you can access it quickly for referring to on those days when you are feeling awful and need to cope. Remember, the goal is to work through it, not suppress it. I know you are probably the *best* at concealing and not feeling, and honestly this is what we women are taught to do, but the truth is that in doing so we are hurting ourselves even further. So grab a pen and paper and make your list. Stop numbing and start working through those emotions!

FULL-FLAVOR LIVING

Chula Story: Mi mami

THIS last chula story is about the person who taught me to *add*. Whether it was sofrito, calabaza, or herbs, mi mami showed me the importance of adding and embracing the foods we grew up with, and it's a lesson I've continued to take with me as a dietitian. This is where full-flavor living comes in. It's about adding the flavors, the sazón, and the nutrition that make us want to eat foods and feel good about it.

Full-flavor living is about doing what you can with what you have while also meeting your health goals. It's not all-or-nothing. It's about personalizing it for you and your family. When people think "addition," they think of adding greens or powders. In a full-flavor life, adding can be quite simple, and this practice was modeled by my family every day, at every meal.

Our meals were complete. Complete meals were important and still are, but they're so different from what American wellness is pushing. For my mom, a dish always had to have a starch, a meat, beans, and a salad. What made them *truly* complete meals was the attention paid to sauces, salsas, herbs, and flavors. It was more than nutrition; meals were to be experienced and felt. Food was about love.

One year when I was a teenager, I was off from school for Holy Week. I accompanied my mom to the many different markets, including Cousins (the Latino supermarket in Philly in the 1990s), for all the ingredients she needed for the traditional dishes she would prepare on Good Friday. I would watch her pick out the chayote, coconut milk, and cod (always purchased fresh at the local fish market). I can still hear her haggling over the price and the perfect cut.

Good Friday is my mom's favorite day to cook; she thrives on this day. We would wake up early and accompany her to the hair salon first. For Good Friday, your hair *had* to be on point. Mine was done straight, and Mami's was flipped. After the salon, we would head home so she could start cooking around ten A.M.

My mami felt so happy to be able to feed the whole family on that day. We all came together in one place to have these dishes that were only made for this day. In this tradition, my mom prepared white rice, guandules, white beans, garlicky shrimp, fried fish, coconut fish, two salads, and of course habichuelas con dulce. Nutrition was never the primary goal of my mom's cooking. She didn't micromanage every nutrient we ate. Like many dishes from around the world, these dishes mean so much more than the individual ingredients. My mom would tell you this labor of love is all about family.

This may sound weird, but the house smelled Dominican to me. The bachata music playing in my mom's small twin-home kitchen—and you can't forget the Jesus episode of *La rosa de Guadalupe* as background noise—transports me back to my childhood. When you'd walk into her home on that day, it felt special.

The house smelled amazing, but you could not pinpoint one specific smell. It was just the overall aroma of these dishes coming together.

Before she would shower and get dressed, the entire table would be set with warm food so guests could eat as soon as they arrived. Think of a big dining room table that seats up to eight people. Mami had the fishes on the far left: a whole fried red snapper (just for the adults because of the fish bones) and the coconut fish, loaded with onions, peppers, and a smooth, creamy tomato coconut sauce.

You'd move down the table to serve yourself the rice, peas, and beans. The white beans were a special request, and I always had more of these than anything else because I would wait all year to eat them. You'd move to the salads next, including a green salad and then a cold, crunchy chayote, zanahoria, and cod salad similar to an egg salad in texture.

Mami's much-loved dish—habichuelas con dulce—is made with a sweet broth, kidney beans, cinnamon, and raisins. At first glance, this would look like a salty dish, but traditionally these beans are topped with small cookies. This is a cinnamony, creamy dessert with just the right amount of sweetness. She would make this dish days before Good Friday, and I can still remember the stacked containers she'd portion out for her out-of-town guests to take home with them. We're talking forty pounds of habichuelas con dulce!

When you think of traditional meals, the assumption is that they are unhealthy and that we should swap in "healthier" ingredients to make them more nutritious. Often, because of the individualism baked into U.S. culture, we feel like our traditional dishes need to be micromanaged or changed in some way. In reality, these dishes do not need to be picked apart, adjusted, or corrected. Yes, even a fish that's fried! It is just one of seven or eight dishes you might eat that day. My mami's traditional dishes for Good Friday are loaded with fiber, heart-healthy fats, proteins, and complex carbohydrates. I want us to go back to a place where we celebrate our roots and traditional foods for what they have to offer.

I have shown you how colonization has stripped us of our land, community, and self-determination, which are integral to our overall health. Now I will show you how to bring them back into your life so you have the tools to experience full-flavor living.

NUESTRA SALUD

A way that I have been thinking about going back to our roots is by looking at how health is defined in Indigenous cultures. In recent years, we have seen a huge decolonization movement around the globe and renewed interest in going back to our Indigenous roots, even though Western medicine has come a long way over the last decade when it comes to lifesaving techniques. And I have become more interested in my abuela's beliefs and teachings about life in the campo, specifically herbal remedies, foods, and wisdom gained from living on Indigenous land. I started reading a lot of books and really connected with the way these authors* saw health. I think it's important to consider how other areas of our lives—not just what we eat—can impact us and how they factor into achieving authentic health.

Indigenous cultures defined health as connection to land, community, and self-determination. It is a beautiful embodiment

---

* Please, porfis, go read two of my favorite books: *The Man Who Could Move Clouds: A Memoir*, by Ingrid Rojas Contreras, and *Family Lore*, by Elizabeth Acevedo.

of the whole self, but somewhere through the legacy of colonization, a lot of that has been lost.

Tierra

Let's consider land. During a time when we used ingredients from our lands, we created amazing, nourishing dishes. These ingredients did not necessarily look like American supermarket buys. Food then meant more than nutrition, it was the fruits of our labor in cultivation and harvesting, and we knew that sustainability was replenishing the land and finding a use for all parts. We created traditions based on holidays and significant events with the foods that kept us going. When we're thinking about food from an authentic place, it's clear that it is made not only to feed you, but also to bring people together. Food symbolizes who we are and how we are connected to the land. When we are disconnected from the land, we are essentially disconnected from our culture—and this is exactly what colonization aimed to do. The juices from our fruta trees, the cilantro garnish from the backyard, and the yuca from the market—all these nutrients serve our health.

The foods and herbs of our land were embraced because of how they positively impacted our bodies, spiritually and physically. Before blood labs and specialist visits, monitoring health in Indigenous cultures was connected back to the frequency and quality of one's poop. The way I look at it, we just need to let go of all the mierda in our lives, and Indigenous practices support this too, quite literally. In traditional Chinese medicine (TCM), it is believed that the small intestine is where we release and clear what is no longer needed in our life. Therefore, having consistent and healthy poop habits represents a broader picture of our health in some cultures, which is why I want to emphasize embracing our cultural foods, specifically our fiber-rich root vegetables such as platanos, yuca, and batata.

We live in a society with a myriad of products that are portrayed as the answer to our health problems, such as having a low fiber intake or digestive issues. You can have both: We can incorporate the foods from our lands knowing they're going to give us the pre- and probiotics to support our digestive health, and we can have fun incorporating the higher-fiber convenient products that can be enjoyed on the go when prep time is limited.

In the United States, we have the ability to practice "both/and" by incorporating a mix of convenient and cultural foods. Unfortunately, when companies occupy our Indigenous lands, such as when McDonald's and Coca-Cola established production facilities in Mexico, they can sell their food products cheaply—but it comes at a cost to the people and their land. The presence of these companies in the Global South introduces a new cultural hierarchy that affects the way people may choose to eat: Eating McDonald's suggests goodness, wealth, and higher status while traditional foods of the land are judged undesirable, poor, and low class.° A hierarchy like this disconnects people from their culture and a traditional understanding of health. In essence, the Americanization of our Indigenous countries has come at the expense of our people and land. One way to reconnect with the land of your culture is to remember a sensory experience related to a time or place where you felt the most in touch with your land.

When I think about connecting with my own tierra, I think of the beach and how healing it feels to me. Ideally it's a Dominican beach, but any one will do. There's such healing for me in being in the sun, with my skin darkening, the warmth of the sun's rays, the

---

° For more context, I encourage you to read *Eating NAFTA: Trade, Food Policies, and the Destruction of Mexico*, by Alyshia Gálvez.

sand in my feet, and the salt water washing away the uncertainties and mala vibras. The beach is where I thrive and feel most alive. Consider this: What's a place that helps you connect with the land?

Comunidad

Connection to the land also emphasizes comunidad. As you know, community is such a big part of our culture, and that directly ties into our health. In our pursuit of the health ideals that we see in the United States and as Westernization creeps into our countries, it's becoming more about the individual than the community. There's a focus on making one ingredient the "hero," while traditional collective approaches to health are being overlooked. Instead of embracing the communal practices that emphasize diverse, shared eating patterns, everything is becoming individualized and reductionist, losing the richness and interconnectedness that has always been at the heart of our well-being.

The lack of community can be seen in what immigrants deal with in this country. When a person crosses that border and enters this country, they are faced with a plethora of issues, beginning with the language barrier and their work status, which directly affect their access to food and the availability of healthcare. We see a shift from community to individualism, from meals to individual ingredients. This shift in particular is notable because it changes the gut flora° of people who immigrate to America. Be-

---

° I met a chula who works at a WIC program office near the Texas border. She sees a lot of immigrants from Honduras who are from the Amazon and don't speak Spanish. They speak Tol, and when they arrive, they often use the WIC program to supplement their purchases of nutritious foods. She described how many of them have gut issues because they are not used to the soy milk and processed foods that are often approved for purchase with WIC funds. They are used to ingredients from the land, and that drastic change has a direct impact on their gut health.

cause immigrants can no longer eat the ingredients of their native lands, their gut flora changes, leading to changes in their health status.[1]

Living within a capitalistic society where immigrants can work the land and feed millions of Americans but don't have access to the fresh fruits and veggies they farm affects Latine health over the long term. They have immigrated to a society where people don't have time to cook, cannot take time off, and live in a vicious cycle of just working to make ends meet. It takes a toll. It can cause trauma, and alter our genetics.

The culture of individualism can weaken our ties with our culture, which is why it's important that we seek ways to find community, whether it's being a part of an inclusive gym, engaging with others in outdoor activities like hiking or birding, joining a group for crafting such as knitting or pottery, or attending local events hosted by your library or in your neighborhood. In Western culture, we have an absence of a "third space," a place outside of home and work. For many, home and work now happen in the same space. Part of our healing lies in finding our third space in communities that enrich our lives and allow us to be more than people who simply work and then get ready for the next day. In a way, this also adds flavor to life.

Self-Determination

And the last way Indigenous cultures define health is through self-determination, which is a lot of what I've taught you in this book, and the key to achieving authentic health. There is not one "right" (ahem, "white") way for us to do anything, especially when it comes to health, which is why I like the Indigenous perspective of looking at our whole self. It's also why throughout this book I've shared information not only about nutrition, but also about how our Latine experience in the United States can affect our health just as much as what we eat.

We can get back to our abuelita's sancocho while also realizing that some of our recipes are very labor-intensive and that there are other ways we can add nutrition. You are not "lazy" if you just need more support in a capitalistic society. You can lean into convenience, you can lean into prepping, you can lean into prewritten grocery lists that combine our recipes and those of other cultures.

We're able to acknowledge the ways in which diet culture has infiltrated our people's lives in harmful ways, and it requires work to undo the conditioning so many of us have been taught. We now understand how to prioritize ourselves when it comes to health—not try to match someone else's strict version of what is considered "healthy." Our cultural foods—while not mainstream—are loaded with nutrition, tradition, and memories. We don't have to be ashamed of them because they don't fit what an influencer online is telling you to eat. As a dietitian, I always heard that these foods were simply loaded with too many calories. Because of the obsession with diets, portion control has become the way that many influencers and even other Latinx dietitians discuss giving ourselves permission to eat these foods. That is, they say that we can have these foods, but only in small amounts. But full-flavor living is not transactional; we do not need permission to eat our cultural foods. We do not need to sacrifice flavor for assimilation.

As a community, Latines face a lot of challenges, and there are many cycles that we must strive to break. While learning how to do so can be a challenge, it doesn't have to be as hard as we think. The way I explain this to my chulas is that we just take it one day, one week at a time. We can always add healthy behaviors and nutrition, and we don't have to do it all at once.

We step toward healing by feeding our panza nutritious foods that allow us to tackle the day. We step toward healing by asking for help and not trying to do it all alone, by giving up the notion that restriction is the only way. We can find authentic comunidad that supports our full-flavor living. We can create a space for a third culture porque somos de aqui y de alla. We don't have to choose. We can always add.

TLDR: Full-flavor living is embracing all parts of your experience: your culture, your preferences, your needs, and your traditions.

ACKNOWLEDGMENTS

First and foremost, to Maria, this book would not have been possible without you. You helped me flesh out my thoughts, you helped me transform all the feelings, thoughts, and education that sometimes are hard to describe, into beautiful words that mean so much. Thank you!

To my kids, Nayla and Brysen, I hope the world will one day recognize us all as equally worthy, and that our differences will be celebrated and appreciated. We are more than enough. I hope you grow up in a world that believes in you. I love you both, all the stars in the sky.

To my husband, Brian, for allowing me to cry, scream, and just go through the motions of writing a book, always reminding me of how much this book is needed. You always lift me up.

To Mami and Papi, who came to this country to give me a better life, I hope I am making you proud.

To my agent, Kate, and my editor, Sydney—Thank you for believing in me. I never thought I would have this chance, and you two really took that chance and gave me this opportunity. When I didn't feel like I was enough, you both told me I was and how much this book is needed. Forever grateful for you both.

NOTES

CHAPTER 1

1. Sylvia R. Karasu, "Adolphe Quetelet and the Evolution of Body
Mass Index (BMI)," *Psychology Today,* March 18, 2016, https://
www.psychologytoday.com/us/blog/the-gravity-of-weight/
201603/adolphe-quetelet-and-the-evolution-of-body-mass-index
-bmi.
2. Adalbert Albrecht, "Cesare Lombroso: A Glance at His Life
Work," *The Journal of Criminal Law and Criminology* 1, no. 2
(1910): 71–83, https://scholarlycommons.law.northwestern.edu/
cgi/viewcontent.cgi?article=1023&context=jclc.
3. Carlos A. Monteiro, Geoffrey Cannon, Jean-Claude Moubarac,
et al.,"The UN Decade of Nutrition, the NOVA Food Classifica-
tion and the Trouble with Ultra-Processing," *International Journal of Epidemiology* 43, no. 3 (2014): 655–64, https://doi.org/10
.1017/S1368980017000234.
4. Ancel Keys, Flaminio Fidanza, Martti J. Karvonen, et al., "Indi-
ces of Relative Weight and Obesity," *International Journal of*

Epidemiology 43, no. 3 (June 2014): 655–65, https://doi.org/10
.1093/ije/dyu058.

5. Frank Nuttal, "Body Mass Index," *Nutrition Today* 50, no. 3
(2015): 117–28, https://doi.org/10.1097/NT.0000000000000092.

6. Huakang Tu, Jennifer L. McQuade, Michael A. Davies, et al.,
"Body Mass Index and Survival After Cancer Diagnosis," *Inno-
vation*, 3, no. 6 (October 2022): 100344, https://doi.org/10.1016/
j.xinn.2022.100344.

7. Perception Institute, "Explicit Bias Explained," n.d., https://
perception.org/research/explicit-bias.

8. M. R. Hebl and J. Xu, "Weighing the Care: Physicians' Reactions to the Size of a Patient," *International Journal of Obesity*
25 (2001): 1246–52, https://doi.org/10.1038/sj.ijo.0801681.

9. Sara N. Bleich, Wendy L. Bennett, Kimberly A. Gudzune, and
Lisa A. Cooper, "Impact of Physician BMI on Obesity Care
and Beliefs," *Obesity (Silver Spring)* 20, no. 5 (May 2012):
999–1005, https://doi.org/10.1038/oby.2011.402.

10. Melanie Jay, Adina Kalet, Tavinder Ark, et al., "Physicians' Attitudes About Obesity and Their Associations with Competency
and Specialty: A Cross-Sectional Study," *BMC Health Services
Research* 9 (June 24, 2009): article no. 106, https://doi.org/10
.1186/1472-6963-9-106.

11. Emile Pereira-Miranda, Priscilla. R. F. Costa, Valterlinda A. O.
Queiroz, et al., "Overweight and Obesity Associated with
Higher Depression Prevalence in Adults: A Systematic Review
and Meta-Analysis," *Journal of the American College of Nutrition* 36, no. 3, 223–33, https://pubmed.ncbi.nlm.nih.gov/
28394727/.

12. Sabrina Strings, *Fearing the Black Body: The Racial Origins of
Fat Phobia* (New York: NYU Press, 2019), 4.

13. Sabrina Strings, "How the Use of BMI Fetishizes White Em-

bodiment and Racializes Fat Phobia," *AMA Journal of Ethics* 25, no. 7 (2023): E535–39, https://doi.org/10.1001/amajethics .2023.535.

14. Susan Dunning Power, *The Ugly-girl Papers, Or, Hints for the Toilet* (New York: Harper & Brothers, 1874), https://books .google.com/books?id=dA8LAAAAIAAJ&pg=PA125.

15. Strings, *Fearing the Black Body,* 124.

16. Sarah J. Hale, *Traits of American Life* (Philadelphia: E. L. Carey and A. Hart, 1835), 165–67.

17. Strings, *Fearing the Black Body,* 209–10.

18. Encyclopaedia Britannica Editors, "Sylvester Graham," *Encyclopaedia Britannica,* July 1, 2024, https://www.britannica.com/ biography/Sylvester-Graham.

19. Elizabeth Stout, "'To Rid Society of Imbeciles': The Impact of Dr. John Harvey Kellogg's Stand for Eugenics," *The Pursuit,* December 12, 2022, https://sph.umich.edu/pursuit/2022posts/ the-impact-of-dr-john-harvey-kelloggs-stand-for-eugenics .html.

20. Anne E. Becker, "Television, Disordered Eating, and Young Women in Fiji: Negotiating Body Image and Identity During Rapid Social Change," *Culture, Medicine, and Psychiatry* 28, no. 4 (December 2004): 533–59, https://doi.org/10.1007/s11013 -004-1067-5.

21. Amy M. Spindler, "A Death Tarnishes Fashion's 'Heroin Look,'" *The New York Times,* May 20, 1997, https://www.nytimes .com/1997/05/20/style/a-death-tarnishes-fashion-s-heroin-look .html.

22. Center for Women's Health, Oregon Health and Science University, "Why Are Eating Disorders on the Rise?," n.d., https://www.ohsu.edu/womens-health/why-are-eating-disorders -rise.

23. Harvard T.H. Chan School of Public Health, "The Economic Costs of Eating Disorders in the United States: Report by STRIPED," accessed September 10, 2024, https://www.hsph .harvard.edu/striped/report-economic-costs-of-eating-disorders/.

24. Marisa Crane, "Challenges in BIPOC Eating Disorders: Prevalence, Bias, and Treatment Barriers," Within Health, accessed September 10, 2024, https://withinhealth.com/learn/articles/ eating-disorders-bipoc-community.

25. "Survey Finds Disordered Eating Behaviors Among Three Out of Four American Women (Fall 2008)," *Carolina Public Health,* Fall 2008, https://sph.unc.edu/cphm/carolina-public-health -magazine-accelerate-fall-2008/survey-finds-disordered-eating -behaviors-among-three-out-of-four-american-women-fall-2008.

26. José Francisco López-Gil, Antonio García-Hermoso, Lee Smith, et al., "Global Proportion of Disordered Eating in Children and Adolescents," *JAMA Pediatrics* 177, no. 4 (April 1, 2023): 363, https://doi.org/10.1001/jamapediatrics.2022.5848.

27. National Association of Anorexia Nervosa and Associated Disorders, "Eating Disorder Statistics," n.d., https://anad.org/eating -disorder-statistic.

28. Flavio F. Marsiglia, Jaime M. Booth, Adrienne Baldwin, and Stephanie Ayers, "Acculturation and Life Satisfaction Among Immigrant Mexican Adults," *Advances in Social Work* 14, no. 1 (Spring 2013): 49–64, https://www.ncbi.nlm.nih.gov/pmc/ articles/PMC3881437.

29. Callister J. Benson, "Acculturation and the Effects on Latino Children's Emotional and Behavioral Well-Being," May 1, 2013, St. Catherine University Library and Archives Digital Collections, https://cdm17519.contentdm.oclc.org/digital/collection/ msw/id/607/rec/31.

30. Rafael Pérez-Escamilla, "Acculturation, Nutrition, and Health Disparities in Latinos," *The American Journal of Clinical Nutri-*

tion 93, no. 5 (2011): 1163S–67S, https://doi.org/10.3945/ajcn .110.003467.

31. "Food Insecurity: Questions & Answers," *Operation Blessing,* accessed September 10, 2024, https://www.ob.org/food -insecurity-questions-answers/.

32. Margarita Alegria, Meghan Woo, Zhun Cao, et al., "Prevalence and Correlates of Eating Disorders in Latinos in the U.S.," *International Journal of Eating Disorders,* 40 (2007): S15–S21, https://pmc.ncbi.nlm.nih.gov/articles/PMC2680162/.

33. David R. Kolar, Dania L. Mejía Rodriguez, Moises Mebarak Chams, and Hans W. Hoek, "Epidemiology of Eating Disorders in Latin America: A Systematic Review and Meta-Analysis," *Current Opinion in Psychiatry* 29, no. 6 (2016): 363–71, https:// doi.org/10.1097/YCO.0000000000000279.

34. Fary M. Cachelin, Virginia Gil-Rivas, and Alyssa Vela, "Understanding Eating Disorders Among Latinas," *Advances in Eating Disorders* 2, no. 2 (2014): 204–8, https://doi.org/10.1080/ 21662630.2013.869391.

CHAPTER 2

1. Abdul Gulloo, "Physiology of Weight Regain: Lessons from the Classic Minnesota Starvation Experiment on Human Body Composition Regulation," *Obesity Review* 22, no. 2 (2021): e13189, https://pubmed.ncbi.nlm.nih.gov/33543573/.

2. Leah M. Kalm and Richard D. Semba, "They Starved So That Others Be Better Fed: Remembering Ancel Keys and the Minnesota Experiment," *The Journal of Nutrition* 135, no. 6 (June 2005): 1347–52, https://doi.org/10.1093/jn/135.6.1347.

3. Sushma Subramanian, "Fact or Fiction: Raw Veggies Are Healthier Than Cooked Ones," *Scientific American,* March 31, 2009, https://www.scientificamerican.com/article/raw-veggies -are-healthier/.

4. Lindsey Haynes-Maslow and Carolyn Dunn, "Low-Income Shoppers and Fruit and Vegetables: What Do They Think?" *Nutrition Today* 51, no. 5 (2016): 242–50, https://journals.lww.com/nutritiontodayonline/fulltext/2016/09000/low_income_shoppers_and_fruit_and_vegetables__what.6.aspx.

5. Feeding America, "Hunger in America," n.d., https://www.feedingamerica.org/hunger-in-america.

6. Feeding America, "Child Hunger Facts," accessed September 10, 2024, https://www.feedingamerica.org/hunger-in-america/child-hunger-facts.

7. Adriane Moreira Machado, Nathalia Semizon Guimarães, Victória Bortolosso Bocardi, et al., "Understanding Weight Regain After a Nutritional Weight Loss Intervention: Systematic Review and Meta-Analysis," *Clinical Nutrition ESPEN* 49 (June 2022): P138–53, https://doi.org/10.1016/j.clnesp.2022.03.020.

CHAPTER 3

1. Evelyn Tribole and Elyse Resch, *Intuitive Eating: A Revolutionary Anti-Diet Approach* (New York: St. Martin's Essentials, 2020).

2. Anjali Prasertong, "The Unspoken History of Early Dietitians and Eugenics," *Antiracist Dietitian*, April 12, 2023, https://anjaliruth.substack.com/p/the-unspoken-history-of-early-dietitians.

3. Association for Size Diversity and Health, "Health at Every Size® Principles," https://asdah.org/haes.

4. Rebecca Stamp, "Average Person Will Try 126 Fad Diets in Their Lifetime, Poll Claims," *The Independent,* January 8, 2020, https://www.independent.co.uk/life-style/diet-weight-loss-food-unhealthy-eating-habits-a9274676.html.

5. Amanda Montell, *Cultish: The Language of Fanaticism,* https://www.goodreads.com/quotes/10960869-modern-cultish-groups-also-feel-comforting-in-part-because-they.

CHAPTER 4

1. U.S. Department of Agriculture, "MyPlate Graphics," n.d., www.myplate.gov.

2. Abigail Tucker, "How Snobbery Helped Take the Spice out of European Cooking," NPR, March 26, 2015, https://www.npr.org/sections/thesalt/2015/03/26/394339284/how-snobbery-helped-take-the-spice-out-of-european-cooking.

3. Ibid.

4. "The ABCs of Nixtamal: All the Vocab You'll Need for Your Kernal-to-Masa Journey," *Masienda,* January 1, 2023, https://masienda.com/blogs/learn/nixtamal-guide.

CHAPTER 5

1. Laura Martinez, "Hisplaining: Why Most Mexican Telenovela Stars Are Güeros," *Hispanic Executive,* March 13, 2023, https://hispanicexecutive.com/hisplaining-why-most-mexican-telenovela-stars-are-gueros.

2. Lisa Kakinami, Bärbel Knäuper, and Jennifer Brunet, "Weight Cycling Is Associated with Adverse Cardiometabolic Markers in a Cross-Sectional Representative US Sample," *Journal of Epidemiology and Community Health* 74 (2020): 662–67.

CHAPTER 6

1. Office of Disease Prevention and Health Promotion, "Social Determinants of Health," Healthy People 2030, accessed September 10, 2024, https://health.gov/healthypeople/priority-areas/social-determinants-health.

2. "Determinants of Health," *GoInvo,* accessed September 10, 2024, https://www.goinvo.com/vision/determinants-of-health/.

3. Sofia Gomez, Vanessa Blumer, and Fatima Rodriguez, "Unique Cardiovascular Disease Risk Factors in Hispanic Individuals," *Current Cardiovascular Risk Reports* 16, no. 7 (June 2, 2022): 53–61, https://pmc.ncbi.nlm.nih.gov/articles/PMC9161759.

4. Genie Kim, Christopher L. Shaffer, Elizabeth A. Allen, et al., "DNA Methylation as a Mediator of the Association Between Stress and Cardiovascular Disease Risk: A Review," *BMC Medical Genetics* 20, no. 130 (2019), https://doi.org/10.1186/s12881-019-0764-4.

5. "Food Insecurity in Latino Communities," *Feeding America,* 2024, https://www.feedingamerica.org/hunger-in-america/latino-hunger-facts.

6. Emily Jensen, "Food Apartheid," Project Regeneration, n.d., https://regeneration.org/nexus/food-apartheid.

CHAPTER 7

1. Lisette Sanchez, "Addressing Generational Trauma and Parentification in the Latinx Community," *HipLatina,* September 29, 2022, https://hiplatina.com/intergenerational-trauma-parentification.

2. Nikhil Kumar, "The Machismo Paradox: Latin America's Struggles with Feminism and Patriarchy," *Brown Political Review,* April 30, 2014, https://brownpoliticalreview.org/2014/04/the-machismo-paradox-latin-americas-struggles-with-feminism-and-patriarchy.

CHAPTER 9

1. Alexandra Bédard, Pierre-Olivier Lamarche, Lucie-Maude Grégoire, et al., "Can Eating Pleasure Be a Lever for Healthy Eating? A Systematic Scoping Review of Eating Pleasure and Its

Links with Dietary Behaviors and Health," *PLoS One* 15, no. 12 (December 21, 2020): e0244292, https://doi.org/10.1371/journal .pone.0244292.

2. Morten L. Kringelbach, "The Pleasure of Food: Underlying Brain Mechanisms of Eating and Other Pleasures," *Flavour* 4, no. 20 (2015), https://doi.org/10.1186/s13411-014-0029-2.

3. Ibid.

CHAPTER 10

1. Pajau Vangay, Abigail J. Johnson, Tonya L. Ward, et al., "US Immigration Westernizes the Human Gut Microbiome," *Cell* 175, no. 4 (2018): 962–72, https://doi.org/10.1016/j.cell.2018.10.029.

BIBLIOGRAPHY

Albrecht, Adalbert. "Cesare Lombroso: A Glance at His Life Work."
The Journal of Criminal Law and Criminology 1, no. 2 (1910):
71–83. https://scholarlycommons.law.northwestern.edu/jclc/
vol1/iss2/6.

ANAD: National Association of Anorexia Nervosa and Associated
Disorders. "Eating Disorder Statistics." n.d. https://anad.org/
eating-disorder-statistic.

Association for Size Diversity and Health. "Health at Every Size®
Principles." n.d. https://asdah.org/haes.

Baier, Leslie J., and Robert L. Hanson. "Genetic Studies of the Eti-
ology of Type 2 Diabetes in Pima Indians: Hunting for Pieces to
a Complicated Puzzle." *Diabetes* 53, no. 5 (May 1, 2004): 1181–
86. https://doi.org/10.2337/diabetes.53.5.1181.

Becker, Anne E. "Television, Disordered Eating, and Young Women
in Fiji: Negotiating Body Image and Identity During Rapid
Social Change." *Culture, Medicine, and Psychiatry* 28, no. 4
(December 2004): 533–59. https://doi.org/10.1007/s11013-004
-1067-5.

Bédard, Alexandra, Pierre-Olivier Lamarche, Lucie-Maude Grégoire, et al. "Can Eating Pleasure Be a Lever for Healthy Eating? A Systematic Scoping Review of Eating Pleasure and Its Links with Dietary Behaviors and Health." *PLoS One* 15, no. 12 (December 21, 2020): e0244292. https://doi.org/10.1371/journal.pone.0244292.

Benson, Callister J. "Acculturation and the Effects on Latino Children's Emotional and Behavioral Well-Being." May 1, 2013. Master's thesis, St. Catherine University Library and Archives Digital Collections. https://cdm17519.contentdm.oclc.org/digital/collection/msw/id/607/rec/31.

Bleich, Sara N., Wendy L. Bennett, Kimberly A. Gudzune, et al. "Impact of Physician BMI on Obesity Care and Beliefs." *Obesity (Silver Spring)* 20, no. 5 (May 2012): 999–1005. https://doi.org/10.1038/oby.2011.402.

Blum, Dani. "Medical Group Says B.M.I. Alone Is Not Enough to Assess Health and Weight." *The New York Times,* June 15, 2023. https://www.nytimes.com/2023/06/15/well/live/bmi-health-weight-ama.html.

Busetto, Luca, Silvia Bettini, Janine Makaronidis, et al. "Mechanisms of Weight Regain." *European Journal of Internal Medicine* 93 (November 2021): 3–7. https://doi.org/10.1016/j.ejim.2021.01.002.

Cachelin, Fary M., Virginia Gil-Rivas, and Alyssa Vela. "Understanding Eating Disorders Among Latinas." *Advances in Eating Disorders* 2, no. 2 (2014): 204–8. https://doi.org/10.1080/21662630.2013.869391.

Cavazos, Emily. "The Inextricable Link Between Anti-Fatness and Anti-Blackness." *ArcGIS StoryMaps,* April 12, 2021. https://storymaps.arcgis.com/stories/11c825a7d1b54829a3056497ad826b4c.

Center for Women's Health, Oregon Health and Science University.

"Why Are Eating Disorders on the Rise?" n.d. https://www.ohsu
.edu/womens-health/why-are-eating-disorders-rise.

DeLisi, Matt. "Revisiting Lombroso" in *The Oxford Handbook of
Criminological Theory*. Edited by Francis T. Cullen and Pamela
Wilcox (Oxford: Oxford University Press, 2012). https://doi.org/
10.1093/oxfordhb/9780199747238.013.0001.

Encyclopaedia Britannica Editors. "Sylvester Graham." *Encyclopaedia Britannica,* July 31, 2024. https://www.britannica.com/
biography/Sylvester-Graham.

Feeding America. "Hunger in America," n.d. https://www
.feedingamerica.org/hunger-in-america.

"Food Insecurity in Latino Communities," *Feeding America,* 2024,
https://www.feedingamerica.org/hunger-in-america/latino
-hunger-facts.

Goldacre, Ben. "How Many Epidemiologists Does It Take to
Change a Lightbulb?" Bad Science, February 1, 2017. https://
www.badscience.net/2017/02/how-many-epidemiologists-does-it
-take-to-change-a-lightbulb.

Hale, Sarah J. *Traits of American Life* (Philadelphia: E. L. Carey
and A. Hart, 1835), 165–67.

Hebl, M. R., and J. Xu. "Weighing the Care: Physicians' Reactions
to the Size of a Patient." *International Journal of Obesity* 25
(2001): 1246–52. https://doi.org/10.1038/sj.ijo.0801681.

Jay, Melanie, Adina Kalet, Tavinder Ark, et al. "Physicians' Attitudes
About Obesity and Their Associations with Competency and
Specialty: A Cross-Sectional Study." *BMC Health Services Research* 9 (June 24, 2009), article no. 106. https://doi.org/10
.1186/1472-6963-9-106.

Jensen, Emily. "Food Apartheid." Project Regeneration, n.d.,
https://regeneration.org/nexus/food-apartheid.

Kakinami, Lisa, Bärbel Knäuper, and Jennifer Brunet. "Weight Cycling Is Associated with Adverse Cardiometabolic Markers in a

Cross-Sectional Representative US Sample." *Journal of Epidemiology and Community Health* 74, no. 8 (2020): 662–67. https://pubmed.ncbi.nlm.nih.gov/32366587/.

Kalm, Leah M., and Richard D. Semba. "They Starved So That Others Be Better Fed: Remembering Ancel Keys and the Minnesota Experiment." *The Journal of Nutrition* 135, no. 6 (June 2005): 1347–52. https://doi.org/10.1093/jn/135.6.1347.

Karasu, Sylvia R. "Adolphe Quetelet and the Evolution of Body Mass Index (BMI)." *Psychology Today,* March 18, 2016. https://www.psychologytoday.com/us/blog/the-gravity-of-weight/201603/adolphe-quetelet-and-the-evolution-of-body-mass-index-bmi.

Kolar, David R., Dania L. Mejía Rodriguez, Moises Mebarak Chams, and Hans W. Hoek. "Epidemiology of Eating Disorders in Latin America: A Systematic Review and Meta-Analysis." *Current Opinion in Psychiatry* 29, no. 6 (2016): 363–71. https://doi.org/10.1097/YCO.0000000000000279.

Kumar, Nikhil. "The Machismo Paradox: Latin America's Struggles with Feminism and Patriarchy." *Brown Political Review,* April 30, 2014. https://brownpoliticalreview.org/2014/04/the-machismo-paradox-latin-americas-struggles-with-feminism-and-patriarchy.

Machado, Adriane Moreira, Nathalia Semizon Guimarães, Victória Bortolosso Bocardi, et al. "Understanding Weight Regain After a Nutritional Weight Loss Intervention: Systematic Review and Meta-analysis." *Clinical Nutrition ESPEN* 49 (June 2022): P138–53. https://doi.org/10.1016/j.clnesp.2022.03.020.

Marsiglia, Flavio F., Jaime M. Booth, Adrienne Baldwin, and Stephanie Ayers. "Acculturation and Life Satisfaction Among Immigrant Mexican Adults." *Advances in Social Work* 14, no. 1 (Spring 2013): 49–64. https://www.ncbi.nlm.nih.gov/pmc/articles/PMC3881437.

Martinez, Laura. "Hisplaining: Why Most Mexican Telenovela Stars Are Güeros." *Hispanic Executive,* March 13, 2023. https://hispanicexecutive.com/hisplaining-why-most-mexican-telenovela-stars-are-gueros.

Montell, Amanda. *Cultish: The Language of Fanaticism* (New York: Harper Wave, 2021). https://www.goodreads.com/quotes/10960869-modern-cultish-groups-also-feel-comforting-in-part-because-they.

Nuñez, Alicia, Patricia González, Gregory A. Talavera, et al. "Machismo, Marianismo, and Negative Cognitive-Emotional Factors: Findings from the Hispanic Community Health Study/Study of Latinos Sociocultural Ancillary Study." *Journal of Latino/a Psychology* 4, no. 4 (November 2016): 202–17. https://doi.org/10.1037/lat0000050.

Perception Institute. "Explicit Bias Explained," n.d. https://perception.org/research/explicit-bias.

Perez, Marisol, Tara K. Ohrt, and Hans W. Hoek. "Prevalence and Treatment of Eating Disorders Among Hispanics/Latino Americans in the United States." *Current Opinion in Psychiatry* 29, no. 6 (November 2016): 378–82. https://doi.org/10.1097/YCO.0000000000000277.

Pérez-Escamilla, Rafael. "Acculturation, Nutrition, and Health Disparities in Latinos." *The American Journal of Clinical Nutrition* 93, no. 5 (2011): 1163S–67S. https://doi.org/10.3945/ajcn.110.003467.

Prasertong, Anjali. "The Unspoken History of Early Dietitians and Eugenics: And What It Can Teach Us About Present Failures in the Nutrition Field." *Antiracist Dietitian,* April 12, 2023. https://anjaliruth.substack.com/p/the-unspoken-history-of-early-dietitians.

Reyes-Rodríguez, Mae Lynn, Hunna J. Watson, Tosha Woods Smith, et al. "Promoviendo una Alimentación Saludable (PAS)

Results: Engaging Latino Families in Eating Disorder Treatment." *Eating Behaviors* 42 (August 2021): article 101534. https://doi.org/10.1016/j.eatbeh.2021.101534.

Sanchez, Lisette. "Addressing Generational Trauma and Parentification in the Latinx Community." *HipLatina,* September 29, 2022. https://hiplatina.com/intergenerational-trauma-parentification.

Spindler, Amy M. "A Death Tarnishes Fashion's 'Heroin Look.'" *The New York Times,* May 20, 1997. https://www.nytimes.com/1997/05/20/style/a-death-tarnishes-fashion-s-heroin-look.html.

Stamp, Rebecca. "Average Person Will Try 126 Fad Diets in Their Lifetime, Poll Claims." *The Independent,* January 8, 2020. https://www.independent.co.uk/life-style/diet-weight-loss-food-unhealthy-eating-habits-a9274676.html.

Stout, Elizabeth. "'To Rid Society of Imbeciles': The Impact of Dr. John Harvey Kellogg's Stand for Eugenics." *The Pursuit,* December 12, 2022. https://sph.umich.edu/pursuit/2022posts/the-impact-of-dr-john-harvey-kelloggs-stand-for-eugenics.html.

Strings, Sabrina. *Fearing the Black Body: The Racial Origins of Fat Phobia* (New York: NYU Press, 2019).

Strings, Sabrina. "How the Use of BMI Fetishizes White Embodiment and Racializes Fat Phobia." *AMA Journal of Ethics* 25, no. 7 (2023): E535–39. https://doi.org/10.1001/amajethics.2023.535.

"Survey Finds Disordered Eating Behaviors Among Three Out of Four American Women (Fall 2008)." *Carolina Public Health,* Fall 2008. https://sph.unc.edu/cphm/carolina-public-health-magazine-accelerate-fall-2008/survey-finds-disordered-eating-behaviors-among-three-out-of-four-american-women-fall-2008.

Thurgood Marshall Institute. "What Is Food Apartheid?," n.d. https://tminstituteldf.org/what-is-food-apartheid.

Tribole, Evelyn, and Elyse Resch. *Intuitive Eating: A Revolutionary Anti-Diet Approach* (New York: St. Martin's Essentials, 2020).

U.S. Department of Agriculture, "MyPlate Graphics." https://www
.myplate.gov/resources/graphics/myplate-graphics.

Vangay, Pajau, Abigail J. Johnson, Tonya L. Ward, et al. "U.S. Immigration Westernizes the Human Gut Microbiome." *Cell* 175,
no. 4 (2018): 962–72. https://doi.org/10.1016/j.cell.2018.10.029.

INDEX

ABOUT THE AUTHOR

Dalina Soto, MA, RD, LDN, is a registered dietitian. Soto is a first-generation Dominican American and she lives in Philadelphia, Pennsylvania.

Instagram: @your.latina.nutritionist
TikTok: @yourlatinanutritionist

ABOUT THE TYPE

This book was set in Horley Old Style, a typeface
issued by the English type foundry Monotype in
1925. It is an old-style face, with such distinctive
features as lightly cupped serifs and an oblique
horizontal bar on the lowercase "e."